The Right to Pain Relief and Other Deep Roots of the Opioid Epidemic

The Right to Pain Relief and Other Deep Roots of the Opioid Epidemic

Mark D. Sullivan and Jane C. Ballantyne

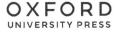

OXFORD
UNIVERSITY PRESS

OXFORD
UNIVERSITY PRESS

Oxford University Press is a department of the University of Oxford. It furthers the University's objective of excellence in research, scholarship, and education by publishing worldwide. Oxford is a registered trade mark of Oxford University Press in the UK and certain other countries.

Published in the United States of America by Oxford University Press
198 Madison Avenue, New York, NY 10016, United States of America.

Library of Congress Cataloging-in-Publication Data
Names: Sullivan, Mark D. (Mark Daniel), 1955– author. | Ballantyne, Jane C., 1948– author.
Title: The right to pain relief and other deep roots of the opioid epidemic /
Mark D. Sullivan and Jane C. Ballantyne.
Description: New York, NY : Oxford University Press, 2023. |
Includes bibliographical references and index. |
Identifiers: LCCN 2022038835 (print) | LCCN 2022038836 (ebook) |
ISBN 9780197615720 (paperback) | ISBN 9780197615744 (epub) | ISBN 9780197615751
Subjects: MESH: Chronic Pain—drug therapy | Opioid Epidemic—etiology | Patient Rights |
Social Cognition | United States
Classification: LCC RB127.5.C48 (print) | LCC RB127.5.C48 (ebook) |
NLM WL 704.6 | DDC 616/.0472—dc23/eng/20220906
LC record available at https://lccn.loc.gov/2022038835
LC ebook record available at https://lccn.loc.gov/2022038836

DOI: 10.1093/med/9780197615720.001.0001

This material is not intended to be, and should not be considered, a substitute for medical or other professional advice. Treatment for the conditions described in this material is highly dependent on the individual circumstances. And, while this material is designed to offer accurate information with respect to the subject matter covered and to be current as of the time it was written, research and knowledge about medical and health issues is constantly evolving and dose schedules for medications are being revised continually, with new side effects recognized and accounted for regularly. Readers must therefore always check the product information and clinical procedures with the most up-to-date published product information and data sheets provided by the manufacturers and the most recent codes of conduct and safety regulation. The publisher and the authors make no representations or warranties to readers, express or implied, as to the accuracy or completeness of this material. Without limiting the foregoing, the publisher and the authors make no representations or warranties as to the accuracy or efficacy of the drug dosages mentioned in the material. The authors and the publisher do not accept, and expressly disclaim, any responsibility for any liability, loss, or risk that may be claimed or incurred as a consequence of the use and/ or application of any of the contents of this material.

For my wonderful and patient family,
Linda, Lena, and Eli

For my parents who took me where I came,
and my husband Stuart who keeps me there

Contents

Preface

We met in 2009, when Mark invited Jane to speak at a University of Washington ethics symposium, "Relief of Pain and Suffering: Too Little or Too Much?", billed as an assembly of researchers, clinicians, historians, and philosophers to discuss the goals, limits, and unintended consequence of efforts to relieve pain and suffering. This was near the peak of the U.S. prescription opioid epidemic, and we were there to consider what went wrong. How could righteous efforts to reduce pain and suffering have turned into an epidemic that had caused so much suffering?

Over the years, we have become close friends and colleagues, written many papers together in medical journals, and spent countless hours discussing the ideas you will find in this book. As we write this in 2021, the opioid epidemic rolls on. In the United States alone, it has cost us 500,000 lives and $1 trillion. The COVID pandemic has not ended the opioid epidemic. Drug overdoses have surged during the pandemic, increasing 30% from 2019 to 2020, up to a total of over 93,000. Overdose deaths from opioids (largely fentanyl) totaled 69,710 in 2020.

Multiple accounts of the origins of this American tragedy have been published. Most of these focus on greedy and duplicitous pharmaceutical companies, flawed drug approval and regulatory procedures, and inadequate scientific testing. Some have focused on the social despair in which opioid use and abuse took root. Our account is different: It will focus on pain rather than opioids themselves.

When patients seek medical help for chronic physical pain, they get prodded and poked, maybe sent for an X-ray or scan, receive a diagnosis, and obtain treatment that could be medication, or injection, or manipulation, or surgery, or physical therapy. All of this can help. Sometimes it can take the physical pain away altogether. Often, however, treatment directed at the painful body part produces only temporary relief. It is the physical pain that will not go away that bothers all of us, because it is this pain that keeps coming back to the clinic, disrupts people's lives, shows up in alarming epidemiological data, and costs society both money and disability. Yet all of this, and the treatment that we aim at it, rarely addresses the personal problem of pain, because it is addressing an impersonal pain signal. This pain signal has been called nociception, or nociceptive input—terms we will use frequently throughout this book. But nociceptive input does not become pain until it has been processed by the person's brain. What the person feels or perceives depends on the person, and can vary dramatically between people and their circumstances, to the extent that for the same signal there could be no pain or terrible pain, or anything in between. This is not a new insight. It has been addressed using behavioral and rehabilitative treatment approaches at least since the inception of pain clinics in the 1960s. But these approaches have been drowned out by medical pain treatments that produce more immediate pain relief. However, these treatments generally leave the person out of the pain treatment process. And when the person's role in the production, maintenance, and termination of pain is forgotten, things can go wrong.

We entered the pain field in its heyday. The idea that pain was not merely a symptom but also its own disease that should have its own specialists and clinics grew out of the birth of anesthesia, attributed to its first public demonstration in 1846. By the 1960s, pain-abolishing treatments were being offered to people with chronic pain. By the 1980s, when we received our specialty training, pain clinics abounded, and there was a belief that new technologies, new techniques, new understanding of pain mechanisms, new medications, and further research would be able to deliver pain relief like we had never seen before. They were exciting times, and pain clinicians were on a mission. Forty years later, however, our high hopes are in tatters. The unfortunate truth is that we have not found better treatments that lower the population burden of chronic pain. In fact, instead of solving the chronic pain problem, it has gotten worse.

The Centers for Disease Control and Prevention (CDC) in the United States declared prescription opioid abuse an "epidemic" in the year 2006. Other wealthy nations face their own opioid problems, though none as grave as those in the United States. Legal cases against the pharmaceutical companies that developed and sold opioid analgesics are in the press almost daily. Many pain medicine professional societies have had to shut their doors because they could not afford the cost of defending themselves in litigation. The professionals and patients who support access to high-tech and expensive pain interventions and to opioids are at odds with those who see these treatments as having low benefit, high cost, and high risk. Instead of rational discussion, they often hurl angry appellations at each other, each believing the other is cruel. At the root of this debate is the right to pain relief through medical care.

This right to pain relief was first established in end-of-life cancer pain care. In the 1980s, palliative care champions argued for extension of this right to patients with chronic pain who did not have cancer and were not dying. In so doing, they were following not only the noble aspirations of the pain medicine movement to control clinical pain, but also the 200-year-old Enlightenment effort to reduce the level of pain and suffering in society to a minimum. These efforts are part of the perennial human quest to control our fate by reducing uncontrolled pain and premature death. This quest has brought successes: Many forms of pain formerly considered to be inescapable (e.g., pain during surgery) are now escapable. This control of pain and death provides some of the clearest evidence of the value of modern medicine and of general progress in human society. Yet somewhere in this effort to control pain we have gone wrong and fallen into some dreadful misunderstanding.

Our modern medical understanding of so-called physical pain as an impersonal, mechanical process portrays pain as something that is imposed upon the person. This pain is believed to originate outside of the person and serves as grounds for the patient's claim to a right to pain relief. Pain is seen as a uniquely medical form of suffering for which it is appropriate to demand medical relief. The right to pain relief provided justification for unprecedented opioid prescribing. It was exploited in pharmaceutical marketing materials devised by Purdue Pharma and other opioid manufacturers that referred to the rights of "legitimate pain patients." We will argue that to end our current opioid epidemic and prevent future opioid epidemics, we must change both our causal and moral pain models.

This book is not a "how to" manual. You will not find within its pages guidelines about how pain should be treated, whether and when to use opioids, which specialist is the right specialist, or what pain services should be paid for. What we hope to convince the reader is that the most fundamental agents of pain management are people themselves. Chronic pain steals away the ability of people to pursue their passions and their distinctive vision of life. Treatment must restore this ability, either directly through restoring these passions or indirectly by modulating the pain experience or both. The person is modulating his or her pain experience all the time. The brain and its internal opioid system constantly adjust our pain experience to promote our survival. We must learn to train and tame this system to our benefit rather than drowning it with opioid medications.

We would both consider ourselves clinicians by profession, researchers and historians by interest. Jane is an anesthesiologist, while Mark is a psychiatrist. Only Mark is trained as a philosopher. We have come to hold similar views on pain and opioids. But our different backgrounds have produced different perspectives and styles that are reflected in the chapters that we each initially drafted. We start off our book with the story of changing beliefs about pain over the centuries. Chapter 1 (Mark) describes how pain changed from being a religious problem into a social problem and then a medical problem. Chapter 2 (Jane) tells of the birth of anesthesia and pain medicine. Chapter 3 (Jane) describes the 20th-century emergence of a right to pain relief. Chapter 4 (Mark) asks: How big a problem is chronic pain? Can we understand chronic pain as a disease? Chapter 5 (Mark) discusses how, despite widespread framing of pain as a biopsychosocial phenomenon, we still see it as an experience with primarily biological causes. Chapter 6 (Jane) describes some of the harms caused by pain's medicalization, where pain relief is pursued by medical and surgical treatments, often to the exclusion of non-medical approaches. Chapter 7 (Jane) tells the story of how opioids were sold and prescribed as specific painkillers in response to the right to pain relief. Chapter 8 (Mark) takes a deep dive into how our causal and moral theories of pain have provided the basis for the claim to a right to pain relief. Chapter 9 (Mark) peels back all the layers we built as this book progressed, reviewing pain as a medical, social, and religious problem. He ends with the question of where pain fits in human life today, and whether the quest to abolish pain has taken us backwards instead of forwards. Throughout, we provide clinical vignettes as grounding for the materials in the chapters. We end with physician and patient epilogues that place the theoretical issues we have raised back into the concrete clinical encounter from the physician and patient points of view.

Our aim in this book is to examine the deep roots of the opioid epidemic that lie in our approach to pain. We hope our book will be of interest to all those people who have been affected by the opioid epidemic and those who are trying to avoid another similar epidemic.

Acknowledgments

We are thankful for the many helpful conversations, seminars, and instructive clinical encounters that we have had with our colleagues at the University of Washington and across the United States. For tolerating our distraction from other responsibilities, we thank our departmental and division administrators: David Tauben, Brett Stacey, Mike Crowder, and Jurgen Unutzer. For reading the entire book, sometimes more than once, we thank John Loeser, Lee Rowen, Bob Kerns, Jeff Fraser, Mike Hooten, Greg Smith, and Lisa Mullineaux. For offering helpful feedback on individual chapters, we thank Judy Turner, Michael Von Korff, Anna Lembke, Fiona Blyth, and Cathy Stannard. We are most thankful to our patients, who have taught us so much over the course of our clinical careers. We are always humbled by their courage, their suffering, and their faith in us as health professionals.

1
The problems of pain
in Western society

Try to exclude the possibility of suffering, which the order of nature and the existence of free wills involve, and you find that you have excluded life itself.

C. S. Lewis, *The Problem of Pain*, p. 25

Introduction: more than one problem of pain in Western society

Pain has always been a problem for Western society, but not the same kind of problem. Until about 1500, pain was primarily understood as a religious problem. Pain and suffering challenged the truth of religious belief and the legitimacy of the Church: How could a just, merciful, and all-powerful God allow so much pain and suffering in the world? As our society became more secular over the next 300 years, pain came to be understood primarily as a social problem. This modernizing society aimed to create the best environment for human flourishing: How might human society be designed and regulated to reduce the pain and suffering of everyone to the minimum possible? At least since 1900, we have separated pain as a medical problem from the remainder of human suffering. We have aimed to reduce this problem to a minimum through medical treatment. This quest has led us to our opioid epidemic. To fully comprehend the limitations of this medical interpretation, we must appreciate how the medical explanation of pain grew out of earlier religious and social interpretations of pain.

Jose Apodaca, part 1

MR. APODACA: This has been a bad year. Six months ago, my wife left me. Now after lifting that box of books at work, my back is killing me worse than ever. I can't work. I can't sleep. I can't do much of anything.

DR. SNAETH: How would you rate your back pain on a scale where 0 is no pain and 10 is the worst pain you can imagine?

MR. APODACA: I don't know. It's got to be at least a 9. It is terrible. The doc I saw in the ED a few months ago when it first got bad gave me some Percocet, which helped me quite a bit, but I ran out of them a few days ago. Can you give me some more of those?

DR. SNAETH (AFTER EXAMINING PATIENT AND REVIEWING THE CHART): It looks like you've had a number of these back pain episodes with a normal physical exam and a normal lumbar MRI. Perhaps we should try some physical therapy before more opioids?

MR. APODACA: I have tried physical therapy. It just made me worse. I need some relief so I can function, so I can go to work. I am going to lose my job at the foundry if I don't stop missing work. Don't you believe I am in pain? Don't you believe I deserve relief?

DR. SNAETH (NOT SURE WHAT TO SAY): OK, I will refill your oxycodone for another month.

This type of clinical interaction occurred many thousands of times at the end of the 20th century. Why did Dr. Snaeth agree to refill the opioid prescription? The answer begins with his acceptance of the patient's claim to a right to pain relief. But this acceptance is based on a great deal of historical and cultural context, of which both Mr. Apodaca and Dr. Snaeth may be unaware. It is based on a notion of pain relief as a reduction in pain intensity. It includes a belief in the privacy of pain and the authority of the patient to determine how much pain he is experiencing. Most basically, it frames Mr. Apodaca's problem of pain as a medical problem of pain reduction to be accomplished using mechanical and pharmacological tools.

Pain and suffering are aversive for individual people. But they also pose a challenge to human meaning, religion, and society. Pain is frightening. It threatens our sense of safety and meaning. It is necessary to expand our perspective to encompass all these problems so that we can place our opioid epidemic in the proper context. This includes looking back before our familiar modern social and medical approaches to pain became dominant. During the past millennium, the problem of pain has been transformed by our cultural context. Before 1500, Christian Europeans lived in a society knitted together by a seamless theological fabric where every event, every fortune or misfortune, occurred because it was willed by God. Everything had a supernatural reason. After 1500, this seamless *moral* fabric was gradually replaced by a seamless *causal* fabric where every event, fortune or misfortune, occurred because it was caused in accord with the universal and unchanging laws of nature. Everything had a natural cause. This shift in explanations of pain—from supernatural reasons to natural causes—is very important for understanding the kind of problem posed by pain and the kinds of solutions offered. But it lies so far in the background of our current thinking about pain that we rarely consider it.

As our cultural context shifted, so did our understanding of the role of pain. Prior to 1500, pain was understood primarily as a moral force, justified for humanity by the Fall into original sin by Adam and Eve, and justified for individuals by their own sins. Pain was present in human life because of original sin and individual sins. Gradually after 1500, pain came to be understood as misfortune that can be causally explained in terms of natural forces and reduced through human effort. With this shift in cultural context, the dominant human questions about pain shifted from "why" questions about the meaning of pain to "how" questions about the mechanisms of pain. Opiates played little role in this shift of cultural context because there was little exposure to opium in Europe before 1500.

Pain as a religious problem

We live in a resolutely secular age, so it is hard to imagine what it was like to live in a resolutely religious age. In his landmark work *A Secular Age*, philosopher Charles Taylor tries to evoke the difference between these ages by asking: "Why was it virtually impossible *not* to believe in God in 1500 in our Western society, while in 2000 many of us find this not only easy, but even inescapable?"[1(p25)] His answer is that we live in a radically transformed cultural context. All our presuppositions about why events occur, about what is to be expected, even about what can and cannot be explained, are different.

By Taylor's account, prior to 1500 European Christians lived in an enchanted world of spirits, divine and malign forces, where everything occurred for a reason. The very order of the world had a transcendent origin in God's will. In fact, God was implicated in the very existence of society. Society existed because of and according to the will of God. Taylor reminds us that the political organization of all premodern societies was connected to, based on, or guaranteed by a faith in God or gods. We are used to thinking of government as having secular origins and justification based on the consent of the governed, as John Locke famously proposed in his *Two Treatises of Government* in 1689.[2] This consent of the governed is mentioned in the U.S. Declaration of Independence. And the United Nations' 1948 Universal Declaration of Human Rights states that "the will of the people shall be the basis of the authority of government."[3] But prior to 1500, government did not exist separately from God and king, nor was society divided into sacred and secular or private and public spaces as is now the case.

The natural world was similarly saturated with acts of God, who was always an active agent in this world. There was no clear division between natural and supernatural worlds. The great events in the natural world— whether storms, quakes, or famines—were acts of God. Everyone felt open to or vulnerable to God and related spirits: Benevolence and malevolence, beyond the human, was present everywhere. In this world, there was no clear division between personal agency and impersonal force. Reasons and causes were not the clearly distinct sources of actions and events that we now take them to be. The human self was porous and vulnerable to spirits and demons and a whole variety of other spiritual influences. This meant that mind and world were not as distinct as we take them to be in the modern era. Sacred objects, like relics of saints, literally contained meaning and power, making sacred healing possible. Moral forces were more pervasive and more important than natural forces. Correcting a moral transgression could correct an illness.

Not only was the enchanted world a different place governed by different forces, but the purpose and goal of life were different. Happiness during one's worldly life was not the goal of human life. Instead, happiness was subordinated to the salvation of the soul and its promise of perfect happiness with God in heaven. Taylor explains that secularized human happiness did not become the goal of individuals or groups for several hundred years. Between 1500 and 1800, Europeans shifted from a sense of human fulfillment inescapably tied to God to one that frequently omitted or denied God. Before 1500, human life was thought to be complete, to make sense, and to be full, only in a space beyond human life. The rewards of virtue and righteousness were not to be found in the natural world, which was fallen and corrupt due to original sin. The rewards of the good life were only realized in Heaven. Pain and suffering in this world served to cleanse our souls of sin and prepare us for eternal happiness. So pain and suffering in this life were not all bad. In fact, they were a necessary component of human salvation. Pain was *not* seen as innocent suffering. Pain was essential suffering because pain supported the moral order of the world. In fact, pain relief was suspect because it might interfere with salvation.

The problem of evil: why does an omnipotent God allow pain and suffering?

Christians believe in a God that is omniscient, omnipotent, and yet is merciful and forgiving. One fundamental challenge, perhaps the most fundamental challenge, to belief in such a God is called the problem of evil. How does such a God allow so much evil in the world He created? How does such an omnipotent God allow innocent children to die prolonged painful deaths from cancer or suffer horrible abuse at the hands of evil adults? This argument from evil is considered one of the strongest logical arguments against faith in an all-powerful God. It is also emotionally compelling. Senseless or random suffering threatens our belief that the world is orderly and that life makes sense.

Prior to 1500, evil and pain were accepted as a necessary part of the moral order of things. They existed because man had betrayed God in original sin and had thus suffered the Fall. This justified, even necessitated, the suffering of humans. On the level of individual human action and experience, illness and sin were inextricably related. Sin sapped our inner strength and made us liable to illness. Absolution from the Church could restore this strength and health. In a world held together by a moral order, sin manifested itself as illness. Pain made sense because it was a punishment for sin. *It was not senseless suffering, nor was it innocent suffering.* Forgiveness for this sin was the path to spiritual and physical healing and to salvation of the soul.

Of course, it was not always apparent to those who were suffering what they had done to deserve such suffering. In the Old Testament story of Job, Satan argues to God that Job is pious only because God has blessed him. Satan predicts that if God were to take away all of Job's blessings, then he would surely curse God. God allows Satan to conduct an experiment with Job where all his good fortune is taken away (Figure 1.1). Job initially accepts that God has taken his animals, his servants, and his children: "Naked I came out of my mother's womb, and naked shall I return: the Lord has given, and the Lord has taken away; blessed be the name of the Lord" (Job 1:21).

As his sufferings mount, Job laments the day of his birth and wishes he could die. Three friends—Eliphaz the Temanite, Bildad the Shuhite, and Zophar the Naamathite—console him, stating that Job's suffering must be a punishment for sin because God causes no one to suffer innocently. They advise Job to repent and plead for God's mercy. But Job's sufferings increase as he is covered with boils from head to toe. His wife urges him to "curse God and die," but he remains committed to God as the source of the world's order and meaning: "Shall we receive good from God and shall we not receive evil?" (Job 2:9–10). As Job's afflictions continue to mount, he accuses

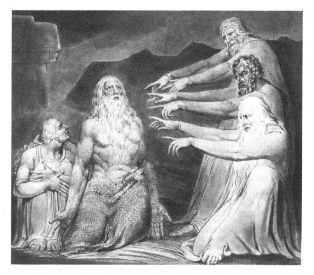

Figure 1.1. *Job Rebuked By His Friends* by William Blake
William Blake, Public domain, via Wikimedia Commons: https://commons.wikimedia.org/wiki/File:Job_Rebuked_by_His_Friends_Butts_set.jpg

God of being unforgiving, fixated on punishment, even hostile and destructive. He accuses God of injustice and abandonment, not only on behalf of himself, but also on behalf of the world as a whole: Why does God not do enough to protect the needy or punish the wicked? God eventually responds, speaking from a whirlwind. But He does not explain why Job is suffering nor why divine justice takes this form. Rather, He reasserts His divine omnipotence: "Where were you when I laid the foundations of the earth?" Eventually, Job admits that he was wrong to challenge God, finally repenting "in dust and ashes" (Job 42:6).

The story of Job makes clear that during this ancient time, God did not simply link illness and sin. Conventional morality in ancient Israel indeed asserted that God rewards virtue and punishes sin. But the Book of Job goes beyond this teaching. The world makes sense only because God created it that way. He alone guarantees that everything happens for a reason. Job ultimately recognizes and acknowledges this. In the end, God restores, and even increases, Job's prosperity in reward.

Job's story can feel very foreign to our modern ear, but it still speaks to us because severe, unexplained suffering still threatens the very meaning of our lives. "Any effective response to suffering must help us recover that meaning," as Viktor Frankl discovered during the Holocaust. "[S]omeone who has a *why* to live can survive almost any *how*."[4(p23)] But explanations of suffering are never complete or completely satisfying. Frankl explains, "No theory or explanation for suffering perfectly accounts for it, and no explanation is universally appealing."[4(p25)] C. S. Lewis offered one of the most famous theories to explain pain and suffering in the presence of an omniscient God when he wrote: "But pain insists upon being attended to. God whispers to us in our pleasures, speaks in our conscience, but shouts in our pain: it is His megaphone to rouse a deaf world."[5(p47)] According to Lewis, pain and suffering are necessary in this world so that we can share a more complete and perfect happiness with God in the next world. In this religious context, suffering makes sense because it is redemptive. It increases our chances of entering heaven.

The most important point for us about Job's enchanted world *is that there was no room for a causal account of pain separate from a moral account of pain. No account of pain's mechanisms was possible apart from an account of pain's meanings. The perspective from which these two accounts could be separated did not exist.* Every account of *how* pain appeared also included an account of *why* it appeared. All forces, natural and supernatural, were personal forces. Pain was essential suffering and could not be understood apart from the person who suffered from it and God who allowed it. Every account of pain assumed the religious function of pain.

Jose Apodaca, part 2

MR. APODACA: Sometimes my pain is so bad that I pray for God to take it away. Or I ask Him why I have this terrible pain. But I don't get an answer. Doctor, do you know why I have this pain?

DR. SNAETH: I think it is due to degenerative changes in the joints and discs of your spine.

MR. APODACA: That is not what I am asking. Do you think I deserve to hurt this bad? Why would God do this to me?

DR. SNAETH: I am afraid that is beyond my training. I only know how to look for causes of pain in your body.

MR. APODACA: Sometimes I wonder if the affair I had last year is the reason that I have this pain. I should not have slept with that woman. It was a bad thing to do, and now I feel that I am being punished.

DR. SNAETH: That does not make sense to me. God does not cause back pain. The causes of pain are found in the body.

MR. APODACA: Of course you are right, Doctor. My brain just plays tricks on me as I try to make sense of all of this pain. Do you think the MRI you mentioned will show the cause of my pain?

Providential Deism: a transitional stage between religious and secular society, 1500–1700 AD

Toward the end of the medieval period, according to Taylor, the nature of faith began to shift toward a more inner and individualized devotion that was separable from Church rituals. Faith became more private and individual. German mystics, such as Meister Eckhart (1260–1328), were important advocates for this more personalized and inward faith. Eckhart, a member of the Dominican order, promoted the ideal of man's self-discovery. He focused on the presence of God in the individual soul. This personal faith provided a response to what was becoming a more private confrontation with death and judgment. But this new, more personal faith still looked to pain and suffering as moral forces that could provide valuable lessons. Eckhart taught that God must be received openly "in oppression as in prosperity, in tears as in joy." Few other great Christian mystics have given so much attention as Eckhart to the presence of God in the painful side of life.[6]

Increased emphasis on the personal aspects of faith coincided with decreased emphasis on the Church-controlled institutional aspects of faith. There was a growing uneasiness with "church-controlled magic." Faith became less focused on sacramental things and, therefore, less "idolatrous." Access to God and holiness became less dependent on the clergy and more dependent on our inner transformation, on "our throwing ourselves on God's mercy in faith." A new educated laity arose to break the monopoly on learning previously held by the clergy. Grace and mystery, especially as these are mediated through relationship with members of the Catholic Church, became less important. This reform of faith looked beyond sacraments and rituals to change the habits and life practices of whole populations. It aimed "to instill orderly, sober, disciplined, productive ways of living in everyone."[1(p244)] This would ultimately lead to the Protestant Reformation and the new idea of salvation through faith. Through faith, individual Christians could gain access to heaven without using priests as intermediaries.

Out of this uneasiness with church-controlled magic, there arose the notion (Deism) of a world designed by God who no longer acted as an agent in that world after it was designed. According to this notion, God created the world and set it into motion, but then did not continually intervene in worldly events. Later commentators would use the "watchmaker analogy" to describe this way of understanding God's involvement with the world: God made the watch (world) and then let it run according to its own rules.

According to Taylor, this "Providential Deism" served as a bridge between a fully religious and a fully secular society. The most important feature of this deism is that it shifts our attention to an *immanent, impersonal* order in the world. "There is a drift away from orthodox Christian conceptions of God as an agent interacting with human life and intervening in human history; and toward God as an architect of a universe operating by unchanging laws, which humans have to conform to or suffer the conse-quences."[1(p270)] God establishes a certain order to things that we can grasp if we are not misled by false or superstitious notions. It gradually becomes possible for human reason to distinguish immanent from transcendent order or, in more modern terms, to distinguish natural laws from super-natural forces.

Most important for our understanding of the problem of pain and suf-fering is that the new order made it legitimate for humans to thrive on Earth, not only with God in heaven. Moral aspiration shifted to realizing the plan God had for us on Earth—"Which means," according to Taylor, "fundamen-tally that we owe him essentially the achievement of our own good."[1(p222)] The faithful are increasingly taught that sin need not be addressed through a personal transformation achieved through the rituals of the Church, but can be addressed as wrong behavior that can be reduced through persuasion, training, or discipline.

This theological shift to Deism is an essential precondition for the trans-formation of pain from a religious problem to pain as a social problem (Table 1.1). It begins the shift from the ancient and medieval focus on "why" ques-tions about pain that seek pain's meaning to the modern focus on "how" questions about pain that seek pain's causes and remedies. With Deism, pain could have natural causes as well as supernatural reasons. It was possible to talk about the causes of pain in addition to talking about the reasons for pain. Pain can now become inessential or escapable suffering.

Pain becomes a social problem in Europe after 1700

> Nature has placed mankind under the governance of two sover-eign masters, pain and pleasure. It is for them alone to point out what we ought to do, as well as determine what we shall do.
>
> Jeremy Bentham (first sentence of his
> *Principles of Morals and Legislation* [1789])

Gradually, it became possible to think of human fulfillment as something that can happen during our earthly lives. Evil was no longer accepted as a neces-sary part of the order of things. This does not mean that some individuals or

Table 1.1 Summary of shifting role of God and pain in the world

	Active Theism	Providential Deism	Utilitarian Secularism
Causation	Active ongoing intervention by God in everyday events; all forces are personal forces	Original order of world as established by God determines events	World has natural fabric of impersonal causation that determines all events
Pain and suffering	Illness and sin are inextricably related; we cannot reduce pain without reducing sin	Pain and suffering teach moral lessons, which individuals can learn	Pain and suffering are natural events that can be reduced without disrupting moral order
Mind and world	No clear separation between mind and world, natural and supernatural, personal and impersonal forces	World has an intrinsic order that the mind can apprehend and anticipate	Mind is independent of the natural world but can know this world objectively
Place of human fulfillment	Justice and happiness are not guaranteed in this world, only in heaven attained through Catholic Church	Individual faith and devotion in this life can earn a space in heaven	We seek to minimize pain and suffering in this world, which is the only world we know exists

sects or denominations will not see pain and suffering as serving as an essential reminder of our need for God; rather, it means that the near-universal consensus about the necessity of evil (in the form of human pain and suffering) begins to break down. It now makes sense to strive for the general reduction of pain and suffering, whereas before this would have been seen as against God's plan for our salvation.

Utilitarianism: reducing pain and suffering as the goal for society

The most well-known and straightforward secular philosophy aiming for a general reduction in pain and suffering in society is utilitarianism. It frames pain as the primary form of evil and aims for its elimination from the world. The first famous utilitarian was Jeremy Bentham (1748–1832,

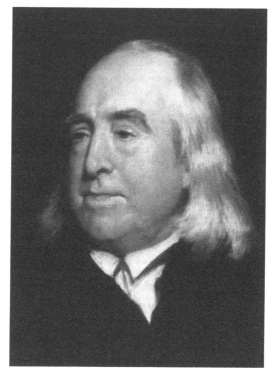

Figure 1.2. Jeremy Bentham
National Portrait Gallery, Public domain, via Wikimedia Commons: https://commons.
wikimedia.org/wiki/File:Jeremy_Bentham_by_Henry_William_Pickersgill_detail.jpg

Figure 1.2), the English philosopher and social reformer who argued for the "principle of utility" in his *Introduction to the Principles of Morals and Legislation* (1789): that the "good" is whatever produces the greatest amount of pleasure and the least amount of pain. "Evil" is whatever produces the most pain with the least pleasure. It is important to note that, for Bentham, these concepts of pain and pleasure encompassed the spiritual as well as the physical. Bentham did not consider physical pain and social pain as essentially different for his theory. He did not separate pain and suffering as experiences with different causes or significance. This difference between pain and suffering will become important only as our social approach to pain and suffering becomes medicalized in the 20th century.

Bentham was interested in applying the principle of utility broadly in legislation, but he was not concerned with medicine or pain care specifically. He saw a society's legislation as vital to achieving the maximum pleasure and the minimum degree of suffering (including pain) for the greatest number of people.

Bentham specified criteria for measuring the extent of pain or pleasure that a certain decision would create. These criteria included intensity, duration, certainty, proximity, productiveness, purity, and extent. He used these to critique policies and concepts of punishment to determine whether an individual's punishment will create more pleasure or more pain for society. He called upon legislators to measure the pleasures and pains associated with any legislation and to form laws that created the greatest good for the greatest number. This legislation needed to be carefully crafted so that an individual pursuing his own happiness would also lead to the greatest happiness for everyone. This was determined through what came to be known as his "hedonic calculus," where pains and pleasures were balanced against one another. Bentham famously argued that these pains and pleasures were not qualitatively different from each other and could be summed up in a simple quantitative calculus.

It is important to note that Bentham's hedonism understands happiness very simply as the balance between pleasant and unpleasant sensations. The one intrinsic good is pleasure; the one intrinsic bad is pain. Although Bentham was sensation-focused in his understanding of happiness, he did not grant the physical sensation of pain any more importance than feelings of grief or despair. Bentham's understanding of utility likely came from Claude Adrien Helvetius's 1758 book *De l'esprit*, in which he argued that humans are motivated only by their natural desire to maximize their pleasure and minimize their pain. Helvetius thus equated morality with enlightened self-interest.[7] Bentham followed Helvetius in that he was a *psychological* hedonist, who believed that all motives for action are based on the experiences of pain and pleasure, as well as an *ethical* hedonist, who believed that pleasure is the only good, pain is the only evil, and only pleasure and pain determine which actions are right.

Bentham's radical ethical innovation was understanding the moral quality of an action completely instrumentally, which means he saw no particular action as *intrinsically* wrong. According to utilitarianism, even lying and murder may be ethical in certain situations. Actions are right or wrong only due to their effects. This denied the longstanding view of the Church that some actions are wrong by their very nature, because they are "unnatural" or violate God's plan. Bentham strongly resisted the idea that he had thereby spoiled or downgraded ethics. As he famously put it: "Is there one of these my pages in which the love of humankind has for a moment been forgotten? Show it to me, and this hand shall be the first to tear it out."[8(p110)]

Nor did Bentham believe, as did other moral philosophers of his time (such as Immanuel Kant and John Stuart Mill) that autonomy and liberty were intrinsically good. He saw these only as instrumentally good. Autonomy and liberty were only good because they tended to increase pleasure and reduce pain throughout society. This hedonic principle extended beyond humans capable of reason to animals. As Bentham stated it, "The question is not, 'Can they reason?' nor, 'Can they talk?' but rather, 'Can they suffer?' "[8(p40)] The capacity to feel pain was more important to ethics than the capacity to choose.

Bentham was also skeptical of natural or universal human rights: "Natural rights is simple nonsense: natural and imprescriptible rights, rhetorical nonsense—nonsense upon stilts."[9(p15)] Rights and obligations were only meaningful for Bentham to the extent that they referred to perceived pains and pleasures experienced by specific individuals. Whether Bentham would have been in favor of a general "right to pain relief" is doubtful. He certainly advocated the minimization of pain through legislation, but he would have seen minimal value in framing this quest in terms of rights. Bentham attacked theologically derived "natural laws" and "moral sense" or ideologically derived "natural justice" or "universal rights" as empty phrases based only on sentiment. By contrast, the utility principle was based on the verifiable material facts of experienced pains and pleasures.

Utilitarianism thus extends the idea that arises in Providential Deism that the order of society should support human thriving. But utilitarianism scorns all reference to divine purpose or salvation in favor of concrete reference to real pleasure and pain. The 19th-century utilitarians followed other 18th-century Enlightenment thinkers in rehabilitating "ordinary, untransformed human desire and self-love." Previously these sentiments were seen to be corrupted by the Fall into original sin. But now, as Taylor explains, "human motivation is seen as neutral; always a mode of self-love, it can either be well directed or badly, irrationally directed. Guided by reason it leads to justice and mutual aid."[1(p253)] Utilitarianism saw "original, unspoiled human motivation as including a bent to solidarity with all others." Secular utilitarianism completed the elevation of reason over grace that was initiated with Deism. It relied more on the integrity of human thought than on the benevolent intervention of God. It broke decisively with the idea that the order of the world had a transcendent origin in God and that this order was primarily moral in nature. *Utilitarianism saw all pain as inessential and escapable.* Human pain and suffering could now become a legitimate target for social reform, and then medical care.

The impartial spectator view on ethics and causality

As Europe became more secular, it abandoned the idea of God as the origin and guarantor of order in the world. However, it did not abandon the idea of a "God's point of view" from which worldly events could be perceived in an unbiased and truthful way. A universalized, disengaged, and objective stance on values (utilitarianism) complemented a similar perspective on facts (mechanistic science). Taylor explains, "Science by its very nature involves our taking an objective, and in this sense universal perspective on things. To see human life in the view from nowhere, or to use a term of the epoch, from the standpoint of the 'impartial spectator,' is to think in universal, and no longer parochial terms."[1(p254)] In both utilitarian ethics and naturalized science, universality and truthfulness is achieved through reason, not through grace or virtue. In other words, in the modern, mind-centered perspective "the physical world, outside the mind, must proceed by causal laws which in no way turn on the moral meanings things have for us."[1(p35)] *From this disengaged perspective, pain does not mete out justice or teach any lessons, it is just evil to be avoided or controlled.*

This disengaged stance toward a disenchanted world is so familiar to us after the Scientific and Industrial Revolutions that it is hard for us to see it. Taylor summarizes, "This powerful understanding of an inescapable impersonal order, uniting social, imaginary, epistemic, ethic and historical consciousness, becomes one of the *idées forces* of the modern age."[1(p289)] We are proud of having escaped from the unreason of the enchanted world. We are proud of our modern sobriety and our immunity to demons.

The disengaged stance recasts the problem of evil but does not make it go away. Severe, unrelieved, and undeserved pain still threatens not only our comfort and happiness, but also the meaningfulness of life. Of all philosophers, Nietzsche probably understood this modern version of the problem of pain the best:

> Man, the bravest of animals, and the one most accustomed to suffering, does not repudiate suffering as such; he desires it, he even seeks it out, provided he is shown a meaning for it, a purpose of suffering. The meaninglessness of suffering, not suffering itself, was the curse that lay over mankind so far.[10(p153)]

This threat of meaningless pain is stronger now that we have stripped away pain's divine meaning.

Modern science and medicine try to solve the existential problem of pain's meaning by solving the practical problem of pain control. We defuse the threat of pain by explaining it and controlling it through impersonal forces. That is why we have gradually and nearly completely given over the problem of pain to medicine and medical science. We rely on medicine to protect us from premature and senseless death. We also depend on medicine to protect us from overwhelming and meaningless pain.

Medicine as the finest fruit of the Enlightenment

From the medieval period though the 18th century, healthcare was more a matter of caring and comforting than diagnosing and treating. Most people did not consult a doctor when they were ill, but relied on brothers and sisters of the religious orders to nurse them in their homes or in hospital wards. Michel Foucault explains, "The nurses responded to the pain, hunger, homelessness, and helplessness of a petitioner rather than to specific medical needs as a physician would. They responded with charity, for their mission was to comfort, feed and shelter, but also to convince and convert."[11(p103)] The public institutions that cared for the ill of 18th-century Paris, such as the Hôpital General and the Hotel Dieu, were not medical in purpose, structure, or staffing. They housed elderly indigents, undesirables, and even criminals who were ailing, but thought incurable. Medical care for these incurables was considered a waste of time and money, so there was one physician, one surgeon, and four assistants for the 15,000 women, men, and children in the whole Hôpital General.[11] These institutions were governed by the principle of charity toward the unfortunate, rather than treatment or cure. As a result, they appeared to be self-perpetuating institutions with an endless influx of men, women, and children seeking admission to overcrowded and filthy wards. One reason these institutions were tolerated was because poverty was thought to be inescapable and a principal cause of disease.

With the declaration of a right to healthcare by French Revolutionaries after 1789, a massive attempt to redirect hospitals from institutions aimed at charity to institutions aimed at health was undertaken. The Poverty Committee of the Revolutionary government wished to disestablish the priority of religion over medicine, and the secularization of the hospital stood as a crucial goal in its deliberations.[11] The new hospitals were to aim at patients' physical recovery rather than their religious salvation. The Poverty Committee argued that the nurse must yield command of the hospital and the patients to the physician and that the requirements of religion be subordinated to those of a scientific medicine focused on disease.

There had been clamoring by organized medicine in France and other countries to reform hospitals according to medical principles for some time. The personal physician to Marie Antoinette, Vicq d'Azyr, wrote in the 1787 report from the Royal Society of Medicine to the Health Committee: "Disease and death offer great lessons in hospitals. Are we benefiting from them? Are we writing the history of the illnesses that strike so many victims in our hospitals? Do we teach in our hospitals the art of observing and treating disease? Have we set up any chairs of clinical medicine in our hospitals?"[11(p169)] After the Revolution, hospitals were investigated and their conditions documented. An effort was made to cull medical problems from general deprivation and poverty, as diseases were considered more amenable to progressive and scientific solution. The hospital now aimed for recovery of the body rather than salvation of the soul, consistent with the general Enlightenment effort to reduce pain and suffering in society.

Health as a prerequisite for happiness

> A practical science is "to be desired … above all for the preser-
> vation of health, which is doubtless the first of all goods and the
> foundation of all the other goods of this life."
>
> René Descartes, *Discourse on Method*[7(p6)]

The modernization of medicine after the French Revolution was inspired by ideas and aspirations developed over the previous 200 years by theorists of the Enlightenment. As the medieval welfare machinery based on Christian charity and hierarchy broke down in the 17th and 18th centuries, a more secular social conscience began to assert itself.[11] Health served as a goal and a guide for these new utilitarian and egalitarian policies as a form of secular salvation. Health was at once a reward for good behavior and a nontheological proof that policies were sound. "According to Thomas Jefferson, despotism produced disease, democracy liberated health. Jefferson believed that a life of political 'liberty and the pursuit of happiness' would automatically be a healthful one."[12(p57)]

For the Enlightenment theorists, the new philosophy and the new medicine went hand in hand. As historian Peter Gay summarized in his two-volume work on *The Enlightenment* (1966, 1969), "It was in medicine that the *philosophes* tested their new philosophy by experience: medicine was at once the model of the new philosophy and proof of its efficacy."[13(p13)] Many of the most notable Enlightenment philosophers, such as Locke and La Mettrie, were physicians before they became philosophers. As La Mettrie declared in *L'homme Machine*, "the great art of healing was man's noblest activity."[13(p15)] René Descartes was not a physician, but saw medicine as man's greatest potential: "All we know is almost nothing compared to what remains to be known; we could be freed from innumerable maladies, of body and mind alike, and perhaps even from the infirmities of old age, if we had sufficient knowledge of their causes and of all the remedies with which nature has provided us."[13(p13)] For these philosophers, reason itself was proved to be trustworthy by its capacity to produce health. Reason liberated us from both prejudice and disease, allowing us to gain control over inessential pain. Even more important, reason would push back the boundary between essential and inessential pain, making what appeared to be inescapable pain into escapable pain.

It is hard to overstate the importance of health and medicine for the Enlightenment theorists. The Christian salvation of the soul was replaced as a social goal by the secular salvation of the body. No longer was it necessary to accept capricious early death as a sign of God's will. Disease need not be accepted as man's fate in an ultimately moral universe. Health was the preeminent social good. It was not only good in itself, but it also enabled all other social goods. Most importantly, as a prerequisite to all public goods, it was not specific to any particular religion or theory of the good life. Health, as something objective, was distinct from happiness itself, but made happiness possible. Objective health allowed for the pursuit of any version of subjective happiness to which the individual aspired. Health was the secular foundation for the good life. As British prime minister Benjamin Disraeli (1804–1881) stated, "The health of the people is really the foundation upon which all their happiness and all their powers as a state depend."[14]

The problem of pain becomes a medical problem

> Our culture—the modern, Western, industrial, technocratic world—has succeeded in persuading us that pain is simply and entirely a medical problem.
>
> David Morris, *The Culture of Pain*

To tell the story of how the enduring, existential problem of pain (in addition to the practical, clinical problem of pain) became a medical problem, we need to reach back a century before the Enlightenment and the utilitarians to the philosopher and scientist René Descartes. Descartes is properly understood as part of the 17th-century Scientific Revolution that thrived a century before the 18th-century Enlightenment. He is important because he applied the new disengaged, mechanical perspective not just to the world, but also to the human body.

During the Scientific Revolution of the 17th century, scientists like Galileo taught Europeans to know the world by disengaging from it and objectifying it using mathematical and mechanical models. This deprived the world of its moral force. It was no longer built by God to prepare us for salvation or to exemplify anything. It did not exist to teach us a lesson. We literally and figuratively no longer stood at the center of God's creation. But Descartes took us farther than Copernicus and Galileo with his mechanization of the human body. Descartes took the human body out of God's world and set it in the impersonal mechanical world. "He calls on us also to withdraw from the meanings correlative with our existence as bodily agents."[1(p285)] According to Descartes's mechanical theory of perception, perceived color is no longer in the dress, nor is the sweetness in the candy, nor the pain in the toe. These experiences are the mechanical products of a world impinging on the body that are experienced in the mind.

After the mechanization and medicalization of pain that follows Descartes, it is no longer possible to read the answers to our "why" questions about pain's meaning and justification directly from God's world. They were no longer written for us there. What could be read from the disenchanted world were answers to "how" questions about pain's causes and remedies. Descartes started teaching us how to find these answers to the newly mechanical problem of inessential pain.

The most interesting thing about Descartes's method is that he built his edifice of knowledge and his mechanical model of the external world and body by first turning radically inward to find a certain foundation for knowledge, famously stating "*Cogito, ergo sum*" (I think, therefore I am). Showing that we could make perfect contact with ourselves through introspection, he showed that the world can run on its own. Descartes thus separated the soul from the world: The soul did not need the world, and the world did not need the soul. Some scholars think this was done to make the emerging natural science compatible with the established religion, by preserving the immortality of the soul and the freedom of the will from the mechanism of the world.

For our purposes, it is important to note that Descartes made pain something extremely inward and extremely outward at the same time. The experience of pain became utterly private and incorrigible, impossible to doubt. Descartes asks in his *Meditations on First Philosophy*, "Is there anything more intimate or more internal than pain?" Yet while he makes the *experience* of pain completely internal to the mind, he makes the *causes* of pain completely external to the mind, in the mechanisms of the body. This is Descartes's famous dualism of *res cogitans* (things mental) *and res externa* (things external). Pain is caused by the mechanisms of the public body, but experienced in the private mind. Despite the implausibility and conceptual difficulties created by this dualism, we are still trapped in it. It separates the bodily mechanisms of pain from the personal meanings of pain. It makes pain the product of mechanisms but not meanings.

As we explore Descartes's legacy, we will draw upon David Morris's *The Culture of Pain*.[15] Although it was published in 1991, before the opioid epidemic began, it provides invaluable tools for understanding the roots of that epidemic in our medical understanding of pain.

Many modern lectures about pain start by criticizing Descartes's famous image of the boy with his foot in the fire from his *Treatise on Man* (Figure 1.3). But Morris helped us see the significance of this image in new ways. The standard critique of this image is that Descartes wrongly implies that the intensity of experienced pain is completely determined by and proportional to the amount of tissue damage produced in the boy's foot by the fire. We now know this is not true: The relationship between experienced pain and tissue damage is highly variable. This is one of the most important and robust findings of pain research over the past 50 years. Sometimes it is added to the critique that Descartes only depicts the afferent or centripetal part of the pain nervous system. We now know that pain-relevant activity in the nervous system flows not only toward the brain, but away from the brain as well. The ascending nervous system that transmits nociceptive information (produced in dedicated receptors and nerves by noxious stimuli) is matched by the descending system that continuously modulates this nociceptive transmission and our experience of pain.

What Morris added to our understanding of this image is how Descartes used it to decontextualize our understanding of pain. Medieval and Renaissance images of persons in pain are rich in context, showing why someone came to be injured or tortured or damaged and what those around him did and felt about this. But Descartes shows none of this. There is no context for the boy with his foot in the fire. The boy is alone with his foot in the fire. We don't know if he was testing himself or tormenting his parents or if he slipped or was forced into the fire. *That is because Descartes is teaching us that we do not need to know these things to understand and explain pain.* What is relevant to the scientific understanding of pain occurs inside the body of the person experiencing pain.

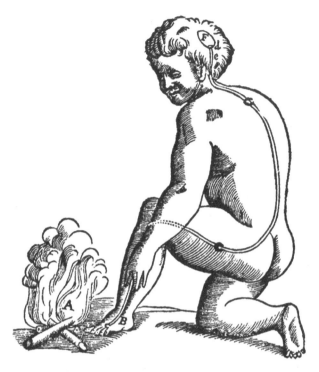

Figure 1.3. Boy with foot in fire, from Descartes's *Treatise on Man*
René Descartes, Public domain, via Wikimedia Commons: https://commons.wikimedia.
org/wiki/File:Descartes-reflex.JPG

By focusing our attention within the body rather than around the body of
the person in pain, Descartes changes the questions we ask about pain from
"why" questions about pain's meaning to "how" questions about pain's mechanisms. Crucially, pain is no longer seen as punishment. There is no role for
punishment in Descartes's image of the boy in pain. The question of punishment no longer arises when the process of pain is depicted like this. Morris
explains: "Today our culture has willingly, almost gratefully, handed over to
medicine the job of explaining pain.... Although almost all eras and cultures
have employed doctors, never before in human history has the explanation
of pain fallen so completely to medicine."[15(p19)] Pain becomes passive and

innocent suffering produced by a mechanical body that is outside the control of the person. *This blamelessness is one of the most alluring aspects of the mechanical medical model of pain and one of the deepest roots of our opioid epidemic.* (There is indeed stigma and doubt associated with chronic pain, especially if it does not have a clear medical cause. We will return to this in later chapters.)

If the medical model of pain is to address the existential problem of pain as well as the practical problem of pain relief, it must make us satisfied with answers to "how" questions as substitutes for answers to "why" questions. Morris explains, "Anyone who has endured a period of intense pain has probably asked, silently or openly, the following incessant questions: Why me? Why is this happening? Why won't it stop?"[15(p31)] We all want pain to stop. But if it does not stop, we want to know why it is not stopping. "Humankind—across cultures and across time—has persistently understood pain as an event that demands interpretation ... It seems we cannot simply suffer pain but almost always are compelled to make sense of it."[15(p18)]

Our increased capacity to control pain that we have gained over the past century or so is surely a great and wonderful achievement. But our ability to control pain through medical means is always partial, never complete. So the "why" questions about pain keep arising. As David Bakan states, "No experience demands and insists upon interpretation in the same way. Pain forces the question of its meaning, and especially of its cause, insofar as its cause is an important part of its meaning.... Its demand for interpretation is most naked, manifested in the sufferer asking, 'Why?' "[15(p34)] This is because pain reminds us we are not in complete control of our fate. David Morris quotes Emily Dickinson's insight: "Pain has but one Acquaintance / And that is Death."[15(p36)] Pain, like death, provides human life its shape and direction. It sets limits on our aspirations and our confidence. If we were able to develop the perfect pain medication, our lives would not be the same. Morris reminds us, "If tomorrow, someone invented a foolproof cost-free pill, with no side effects, guaranteeing life-time immunity from pain, we would at once have to set about reinventing what it means to be human."[15(p20)] Human life is framed by death and by pain. Without this frame, we would not recognize it.

Physical versus mental pain

One of the ways that our culture makes the mechanical understanding of pain plausible and acceptable is by dividing physical pain, caused by tissue injury inside the body, from mental or psychological pain, caused by social injury outside the body. We don't just distinguish the causes of these types of pain, but we also value them differently in our medical perspective. Pain associated with visible injury is real pain. This is literal pain. Pain associated with abandonment or exclusion or neglect is less real pain. It is only pain in a metaphorical sense. David Morris has referred to this as the "Myth of Two Pains": "You feel physical pain if your arm breaks, and you feel mental pain if your heart breaks."[15(p9)] We did not always separate pains in this way. The English word "pain" is derived from the Middle English *pane* and the French *peine,* which mean "punishment; penalty; suffering or loss inflicted for a crime or offence."[16] Neither the medieval nor the Enlightenment thinkers we discussed above made this distinction between physical and mental pain. In ancient Greece, Aristotle treated pain like an emotion, similar to joy.

It is with Descartes that we get a concept of pain as a sensation produced mechanically by bodily injury. The body registers tissue damage and transmits this information through nerves and spinal cord to the brain. The pineal gland is where the mechanical body interacts with the sentient mind, producing the sensation of pain. But Descartes did not strongly distinguish the production of sensory sensations like pain from the production of emotions, which he referred to as passions. In his final philosophical treatise, *The Passions of the Soul* (1649), Descartes defines the passions as "the perceptions, sensations, or commotions of the soul which we relate particularly to the soul and are caused, maintained, and strengthened by some movement of the spirits."[17(p27)] These "spirits" are "animal spirits," which are produced in the blood and "move the body in all the different ways it is capable of." Although Descartes espouses a strong dualism of mind and body, he saw both sensations and emotions as mechanical productions of the body that were imposed on the mind. He argued that there were only six distinct passions: wonder, love, hatred, desire, joy, and sadness. All other passions were formed as combinations or subtypes of these.

Thus, our contemporary distinction between physical and mental pain cannot be attributed to Descartes. Rather, this opposition has evolved out of the culture of modern biomedicine that looks for the cause of subjective symptoms in objective disease. But what mental or psychogenic pain means is not clear. Sometimes "mental pain" refers to anguish or despair that is not experienced as arising from a body location. Yet this pain can be very significant as it can prompt a desire to die or a suicide attempt. Other times "mental pain" refers to pain of social origin that is experienced as having a bodily location and possibly a bodily cause. Sometimes this is called psychogenic pain. Chest pain after experiencing a catastrophic loss of a loved one would be one example. Another example would be headaches that occur in conjunction with a major depressive episode. Often, psychogenic pain remains a diagnosis of exclusion, meaning that pain without identifiable physical cause is labeled as psychogenic without independent evidence of a psychological cause. For example, in 1967 pain experts Merskey and Spear defined psychogenic pain as "pain which is independent of peripheral stimulation or of damage to the nervous system and due to emotional factors, or else pain in which any peripheral change (e.g., muscle tension) is a consequence of emotional factors."[18(p17)] This suggests that diagnoses of mental or psychogenic pain are not diagnoses with clear positive criteria. Since they essentially rely on the exclusion of physical causes for pain, they are actually diagnoses of "not-physical pain." This can imply that pain without identifiable objective cause is "unreal pain," a label that all patients with chronic pain fear and loathe.

Origin of physical versus mental pain dichotomy in the diagnosis of objective disease

To understand how we have come to divide physical from mental pain, we must review how physicians began to diagnose objective disease. Michel Foucault has described in his *Birth of the Clinic* how fully objective access to the patient's disease was achieved in Paris around 1800. Up until 1800, diseases were perceived, defined, and classified into botanical families according to symptoms experienced by the patient. These diseases of experienced qualities were perceived most clearly and naturally in the patient's home. Disease could be seen clearly in the home and was only distorted by the artificiality of the hospital.[11] The study of epidemics served as a transition between the 18th-century medicine of the patient's home and the 19th-century medicine of the hospital. "The need to control epidemics introduced medicine to a collective, open consciousness of the series of cases."[11(p27)] Epidemic surveillance introduced a new form of observation into medical practice that was less individualized and less personal. It allowed doctors to begin to see the "same" disease in very different patients. Now, both the serf and the priest could be diagnosed with the same hepatitis. This new perspective separated diagnosis from biography, and disease from person.

This surveillance of cases in epidemics made it possible for physicians to see a series of diseases appearing in patients, rather than a series of unique patients afflicted with personal diseases. But the ultimate laboratory for this type of impersonal observation was the modern hospital rather than the patient's home. This new setting redefined what was "signal" and what was "noise" for clinical observation. The signal was what could be observed about the disease as the patient lay in a hospital bed. The noise was details of the patient's life and biography that were more apparent in his own home. The hospital thus provided both a uniform place of discovery and a novel logic of discovery for medical facts. This place was to become the home of both medical teaching and research. It is where modern disease and pain are defined.

Once observation of patients in their beds is established as the canonical form of clinical observation, the stage is set for the clinico-pathological correlation of these clinical findings with those of patients' organs on the autopsy table—as Foucault phrases it, "an objective, real, and at last unquestionable foundation for the description of diseases."[11(p27)] Disease classification and diagnosis were no longer tied to categories based in patients' experience, but could be based on the correlation between observed clinical signs and observed pathological lesions at autopsy. Uncertain clinical diagnosis could be definitively corrected through this process of clinico-pathological correlation. Disease was thus no longer most accurately perceived from *within* the life afflicted, but observed from *outside* that life through the lens of death provided by the autopsy. The autopsy became the definitive way to know disease, eclipsing all patient accounts of disease experience. Practical innovations that allowed dissection to occur close to the time of death, like autopsy rooms close to hospital rooms, permitted death to be a clear window on disease. Death now opened the body and its diseases to observation, rather than obscuring them under the gray cloud of decay.

Death is thus remarkably transformed from a source of distortion in clinical perception into the privileged point of view on disease. With death revealing the pathological lesion as the finally visible core of the disease, the clinical interpretation of signs and symptoms shifts. Signs and symptoms no longer point to each other within the life of the patient, but point outside that life experience to the objective tissue lesion that defines and causes the disease. Clinical and laboratory examinations of the living patient now anticipate and are corrected by the autopsy examination. The patient's subjective experience of disease is no longer essential to the medical diagnosis of disease.

Disease and health can now be fully objective. The physician, bolstered by medical tests, will now hold final authority about whether disease is present and whether health care is needed. *Pain is no longer an essential component of disease definition and experience, but merely a symptom of a disease defined as tissue damage.* This is the beginning of the distinction between "physical" (meaning verifiably medical pain) and "non-physical" pain. Real physical pain is pain caused by objective tissue damage. It is this pain that is of medical importance and therefore clinical concern. It may offer crucial information about how to save the patient's life, unlike "non-physical" pain.

Jose Apodaca, part 3

MR. APODACA: This back pain is so bad, something must be broken in there. If we could only find it and fix it, I would be alright. My neighbor says they missed the slipped disc in his back for years. I don't want to just take pills, I want to find out what is wrong with my back.

DR. SNAETH: I don't see any worrisome danger signs that something serious is causing your back pain. But it has been going on a long time now, and it's getting worse, so I think we can get another MRI.

MR. APODACA: That will really help. My employer does not understand why I am not coming back to work. If I had a picture to show him, he would understand. I think he thinks I am making all this up, or exaggerating the pain. I know my pain is real but he doesn't.

The emergence of a right to health and healthcare

The right to pain relief must be understood within the history of the rights to health and healthcare. As economies shifted from a feudal to mercantile basis at the end of the medieval period, trading gave rise to larger cities. This urbanization gave rise to a new type of concern about public health. Historian Dorothy Porter explains that concerns with health in this period began to focus less on the comfort of elites and more upon the contagious diseases of the poor. In the city, the diseased poor were a more concrete threat to the health of elites and, thus, became the focus of more attention and regulation.[12] With further urbanization, the nature of the infections that posed a threat to public health also began to shift. By the 18th century, epidemics were being replaced as the primary public health concern by high levels of endemic infections and chronic illness, such as malaria, smallpox, and gout.[12] Intermittent concern about epidemics gave way to a continuing concern about the high rate of endemic infections in vulnerable urban populations, such as among infants and children. Newly centralized governments developed strategies for monitoring the public health of their populations. Mortality and morbidity rates began to be calculated, as indices of national health.

Medical criteria and categories also gained prominence in every aspect of the hospital. The hospital admitting office "practiced stern medical triage: malingerers (*faux malades*) now found themselves blacklisted."[19(p11)] Only those patients with legitimate and verifiable medical conditions were admitted to the hospital. Physicians learned from surgeons how to validate symptom reports by reference to observed signs such as edema, fever, and rash, or to signs elicited with the palpating hand on liver, stomach, or spleen. Instruments that allowed observation to penetrate the body (thus anticipating the autopsy), such as the stethoscope, came later. Doctors were now allowed to prioritize patients for admission based on their value for medical education. This medical hospital acquired the authority to select its patients and to admit only those with legitimate diseases (e.g., not "interminable chronic complaints"). Patients were arranged so their diseases could best be observed. "Place hospital patients so that the sequence of their beds represents ... the thermometer of seriousness of their diseases," stated C. F. Duchanoy, MD, in 1801.[19(p166)] In return for their free care, charity patients were expected to submit to repeated examination and probing to identify disease by doctors and student doctors. After death, their families were expected to allow dissection at autopsy. It was the autopsy that corrected the clinical diagnosis of disease and ultimately guaranteed its objectivity.

As French patients shifted from being the "ailing poor" of the old regime to citizens with a right to healthcare at the beginning of the 19th century, the social position of the medical profession also shifted. In accord with the ideals of the Revolution, François, duc de La Rochefoucauld-Liancourt, proposed that citizens have "prompt, free, assured and complete" healthcare.[11] But such an absolute right would bankrupt any modern society, so it became necessary to regulate and restrict this right to healthcare. One of the first places this was done was at the door to the hospital. Because medical criteria were now used to determine whether someone was admitted to the hospital or other medical services, physicians gained more social power as gatekeepers. Foucault explains, "It was the doctor who discovered where [assistance] was needed and judged the nature and degree of the assistance to be given.... In addition to his role as a technician of medicine, he would play an economic role in the distribution of help, and a moral, quasi-judicial role in its attribution; he would become 'the guardian of public morals and public health alike.'"[11(p41)] Physicians gained control over the definition of health and over who needed healthcare. Physicians similarly gained power to validate pain complaints as physical or legitimately medical, or invalidate them as "mental" or "psychological" and, therefore, not legitimately medical. Patient claims to a right to pain relief made since the 1990s have especially focused on pain validated as physical. Purdue Pharma regularly referred to these as "legitimate pain patients."

Conclusion: the problems of pain, from religious to social to medical framing

The problem of pain has taken many forms over the last millennium, culminating with a contemporary claim to a right to medical pain relief, endorsed by both patients and professional organizations. We have described the religious approach to pain as prevalent until 1500, with a transitional period of Deism between 1500 and 1700. This approach saw pain and suffering as a form of evil that threatened faith and meaning. As society secularized after 1700, a social approach to the problem of pain became dominant. In this period, pain ceased to be evidence of an evil force or of limitations to God's power and became synonymous with evil itself. Utilitarians stated it most clearly: Pain is bad/evil, and pleasure is good. They attempted to erase our understanding of any pain as essential or inescapable, portraying all pain as inessential or escapable. The social good was to reduce pain and suffering as much as possible, but the utilitarians did not separate pain from the rest of human suffering. This would only happen as pain was approached as a medical problem.

Around 1800, professional medicine began to pull away from other social welfare efforts to focus on the treatment of objective disease. Gradually, pain associated with objective disease also became a focus of medical diagnosis and treatment. Pain was separated from the rest of human suffering as the product of objective disease. Pain not clearly associated with verifiable disease or damage is not so important for a medicine focused on preventing premature death. Pain that is not caused by disease or damage becomes a distinct domain of mental or psychological pain, which is treated as a private or personal concern, not a responsibility of the professional medical system. Religious and social means of addressing the problem of pain do not disappear in modern society but become marginalized in favor of the medical approach. Now, a general right to pain relief through the medical reduction of pain intensity makes sense.

In the past 35 years, we have turned to opioid medications at an unprecedented level in the effort to take control of our pain and our lives. As that effort has spun out of control into our current opioid epidemic, we must ask: What went wrong? In this book, we argue that we have misunderstood not only the tool of opioids, but the goal of pain control. We have separated pain from the rest of human suffering as a uniquely mechanical and medical affliction. This scientific framing of pain as due to impersonal mechanical forces has facilitated a moral framing of pain as passive and innocent suffering. Once pain is framed in this way, the right to pain relief makes sense. Patients, like Mr. Apodaca, did claim this right to pain relief from their primary care providers in the form of opioid prescriptions.

References

1. Taylor C. *A Secular Age*. Harvard University Press; 2007.
2. Locke J. *Two Treatises of Government*. Cambridge University Press; 1988 (first published in 1689).
3. United Nations. *Universal Declaration of Human Rights*. 1948. https://www.un.org/en/about-us/universal-declaration-of-human-rights
4. Rice R. *Suffering and the Search for Meaning: Contemporary Responses to the Problem of Pain*. InterVarsity Press; 2014.
5. Lewis CS. *The Problem of Pain*. Harper Collins; 2001.
6. Meister Eckhart. 2011. https://en.wikipedia.org/wiki/Meister_Eckhart
7. Helvetius CA. *De l'ésprit, or, Essays on the Mind and Its Several Faculties*. B. Franklin; 1970 (first published in 1758).
8. Bentham J. *An Introduction to the Principles of Morals and Legislation*. Clarendon Press; 1789.
9. Bentham J. *Anarchical Fallacies: Being an Examination of the Declaration of Rights Issued During the French Revolution. Nonsense upon Stilts*. Routledge; 1789.
10. Nietzsche F. *The Genealogy of Morals*. Random House; 1967 (first published in 1887).
11. Foucault M. *The Birth of the Clinic: An Archeology of Medical Perception*. Vintage Books; 1973.
12. Porter D. *Health*, Civilization, and the State: A History of Public Health from Ancient to Modern Times. Routledge; 1999.
13. Gay P. *The Enlightenment: An Interpretation*. Knopf; 1969.
14. Benjamin Disraeli. Wikipedia; 2020. https://en.wikipedia.org/wiki/Benjamin_Disraeli
15. Morris D. *The Culture of Pain*. University of California Press; 1991.
16. Oxford English Dictionary. 2005. https://www.oed.com/
17. Descartes R. *Passions of the Soul*. Earlymoderntexts.org; 2010 (first published in 1669). https://www.earlymoderntexts.com/authors/descartes
18. Merskey H, Spear FG. *Pain: Psychological and Psychiatric Aspects*. Bailliere, Tindall & Cassell; 1967.
19. Weiner D. *The Citizen-Patient in Revolutionary and Imperial Paris*. Johns Hopkins University Press; 1993.

2
The medical dream of conquering pain

On October 16, 1846, William T. G. Morton, a Boston dentist, publicly demonstrated the removal of a tumor under ether anesthesia in a lecture theater in Massachusetts General Hospital. The event caught the world's imagination. "We have conquered pain" was the cry spread by the press all around the globe. In fact, neither ether nor painless surgery was new, but then, as Sir William Osler said when presenting Morton's original paper to London's Royal Society of Medicine in 1918: "In science, the credit goes to the man who convinces the world, not to the man to whom the idea first occurs."[1]

It is easy to understand public exuberance at the notion that pain could be controlled. Along with preventing premature death, it is a core component of controlling our fate on this earth. Medicine helps identify our afflictions through diagnosis, predict their future course through prognosis, and reduce their effects on our lives through therapy. In addition to diagnosing and curing disease, modern medicine has helped reduce the pain associated with our vulnerability to death and disease.

This control over disease and pain is one of the finest fruits of the Scientific Revolution and of the modern biomedicine that grew out of it. It has helped us overcome the fatalism of the Middle Ages and instilled us with confidence and ambition about reducing the total amount of pain and suffering in society. It has shifted the boundary between pain that we must accept and pain that we can relieve.

Julia Arnold, part 1

Julia Arnold (b. 1944) was a teenager when she first complained of abdominal pain. The pain was so bad that she sometimes missed school for days at a time. When she had a period, the pain was worse, but the pain was not limited to menstruation. She underwent a battery of tests over several years, but nothing could be found to explain her abdominal pain. At the suggestion of a friend, she came to you for diagnosis and treatment of her pain. On abdominal and pelvic exam, you think you feel a mass. You order an ultrasound that demonstrates an ovarian cyst. The cyst was not huge (about 4 cm), but you think it might be causing the pain and suggest that it be removed. Julia undergoes a laparotomy under general anesthesia to remove her cyst. She awakens the next morning with surgical pain, but without her crampy abdominal pain. As her surgical pain resolves, she is pain-free for the first time in years.

Though the birth of modern anesthesia did not conquer pain, it did change the way we think about pain. Pain during surgery was no longer inevitable; suddenly there was a means of subsuming it under a blanket of insensibility. In fact, all that had occurred was the perfecting of techniques to deliver measured amounts of anesthetic vapors so that these agents could be delivered relatively safely. Opium and alcohol had been used for millennia to produce insensibility and, thus, reduce pain temporarily, so there was nothing new about using vapors and many other toxins to induce insensibility. The breakthrough was to be able to do it safely and reversibly. The importance of Morton's demonstration was that it opened up the new field of anesthesia, the achieving of insensitivity to pain during surgery.

This medical breakthrough had significance beyond the practice of medicine. To make this significance clear, we draw upon a distinction made by Martin Luther in the 1500s about suffering and discussed recently by Tanya Luhrmann in relation to mental illness.[2] Luther defines the distinction between essential (or inescapable) suffering and inessential (or escapable) suffering. Luther's approach to suffering does not strongly distinguish between pain and suffering, which will come later, as the medical approach becomes dominant.

Essential suffering is what we are not able to prevent but must survive if we can. Essential suffering is the inherent difficulty of human life, our troubles, the way we struggle in the world, being the specific people we are, of a certain character, in this specific place and time. The particular history of our pain molds our characters further into the people we become. Human pain is inevitable, and all the knowledge and fervor in the world will not wash it away safe and pure.[2(p272)]

Prior to surgical anesthesia, the pain of surgery, like the pain of dying, was seen as inescapable, essential suffering. After the demonstration of safe and effective surgical anesthesia, it became escapable, inessential suffering. What had been deeply accepted as uncontrollable was revealed as controllable, and not through virtue or prayer, but scientific technique. With anesthesia, surgical pain became inessential suffering.

> Inessential suffering is the pain we can treat. We can remove it because it is the result of some fact that can be altered. When it is gone, it is inessential to us. It has not made us who we are. Luther argues that illness that can be cured, hunger that can be fed, and chill that can be warmed are inessential sufferings, and it is our duty to remove them.[2(p272)]

According to Luhrmann, in our culture, "medicine handles the inessential suffering and religion handles the essential suffering."[2(p272)] Thus, safe and effective anesthesia shifted surgical pain from the domain of religion into the domain of medicine. The stage was set for someone to try to shift other forms of pain from the inescapable category to the escapable category through the application of medical expertise.

John Bonica and the founding of pain medicine

Given the magnitude of the breakthrough brought about by the birth of anesthesia in terms of reducing human suffering, perhaps it is not surprising that the next great breakthrough in the control of pain came from an anesthesiologist, John Bonica. Born in Sicily in 1917, the oldest child of the local director of postal services and his wife, a midwife, John Bonica became fascinated with medicine as he watched his mother on her rounds. The family immigrated to the United States in 1928, seeking better opportunities for the children. But tragedy struck the family in 1932 when Bonica senior died at only 55, leaving the family with meager savings. John Bonica felt responsible for his family and put his considerable strength and determination into studying and earning income. He became a professional wrestler, achieving the title of Light Heavyweight Champion of the World in 1941, an early mark of the man. Despite the rigors of professional wrestling, he continued his education, fulfilled his childhood ambition to become a physician, and graduated from medical school in 1942. He also married in 1942, and when his wife suffered a near-fatal anesthetic mishap the following year during childbirth (from which he saved her), he determined to enter the field of anesthesia. By 1944, he had completed anesthesia training and quickly became one of the most highly regarded and influential anesthesiologists in the United States (Figure 2.1).

Another significant development in the years between the birth of anesthesia and John Bonica's adoption of that specialty was the recognition that cocaine, which had previously been known to have numbing effects only

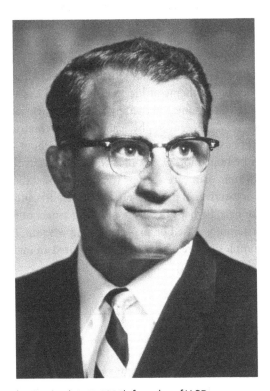

Figure 2.1. John Bonica (1917–1994), founder of IASP
Permission obtained from Wood Library—Museum of Anesthesiology

on mucosae, could be injected around nerves to produce regional anesthesia. This led rapidly to the formulation of other, safer local anesthetics, and by the end of the 19th century, blockade of every nerve in the body had been described. By the time John Bonica adopted anesthesia as his passion in 1944, regional anesthesia had gained equal prominence with general anesthesia for surgical use. These two branches of surgical anesthesia rotated in popularity according to which anesthetic disaster was more recent!

Because of his wife's near-fatal obstetric anesthesia mishap, Bonica started his anesthesia career specializing in obstetric anesthesia. Here, he helped improve the techniques of epidural, spinal, and field anesthesia for childbirth, which were in their infancy at the time. The success of regional anesthesia for the pain of labor and delivery helped ignite the idea that nerve-blocking techniques could relieve chronic pain, not just pain from critical events. Bonica himself struggled with chronic back pain brought about by many years of professional wrestling. Even though Bonica's personal interest and skill lay in anesthetic techniques for the relief and diagnosis of pain, he recognized that chronic pain therapy needed to reach beyond nerve blocks and other anesthetic techniques. Although analgesic blocks were the central theme of his 1953 textbook, *The Management of Pain*, he recognized that physical therapy and psychiatric techniques were often also necessary: "Moreover, physical and/or psychiatric therapy constitute integral phases in the management of pain without which optimal results cannot be hoped for."[3(p6)] Bonica was the first advocate for multidisciplinary chronic pain care—a new treatment model that would bring together the perspectives of multiple medical specialists and nonphysician health professionals. Perhaps the most enduring aspect of Bonica's legacy was his understanding, based on experience and wisdom, that the multifaceted and complex nature of chronic pain required an integrated, multifaceted management strategy.

Julia Arnold, part 2

After a few pain-free years, Julia begins having some abdominal pain during menstruation again. She has graduated from high school, and trained to be a hairdresser. At 24, she is unmarried, shares an apartment with two girlfriends, works as a hairdresser, and presents to you again because her abdominal pain has begun to interfere with her life again.

A pelvic exam and an ultrasound are unable to identify any ovarian cyst. She is sent home with reassurance that she does not have another ovarian cyst. However, she continues to have abdominal pain with menstruation and she returns for care a few months later. A repeat ultrasound again fails to find a sizeable ovarian cyst but suggests that there might be cystic endometriosis on her bowel. A consulting OB-GYN suggests laparoscopic surgery to diagnose and, if needed, to treat endometriosis. Laparoscopy under general anesthesia does show some small areas of endometriosis on the wall of the sigmoid colon; they are partially removed and partially cauterized.

Julia recovers from the surgery without problems. Unfortunately, she does not get lasting pain relief from the surgery. You decide to send her to the new pain clinic that had opened in your town. They administer a superior hypogastric nerve block with local anesthetic and steroid. Over the next few months she reports significantly less pain during her periods. She is now able to work through her pain episodes.

John Bonica is credited with being the founding father of pain medicine. With the rise of pain medicine, chronic pain would become a disease in its own right, with its own specialists and its own clinics. Bonica recognized that pain's complexity required more than one expert or one specialty to manage it. That insight led to the first multidisciplinary pain clinic in Tacoma, Washington, where he was chief of anesthesia during the post-WWII years. In 1960, he moved to the University of Washington in Seattle and founded its Department of Anesthesia and its multidisciplinary pain center. By the late 1970s, over 170 clinics had been developed in the United States on the Bonica multidisciplinary model. Interestingly, during Bonica's career, psychological and regional surgical approaches to chronic pain were emphasized in the multidisciplinary clinics, along with drug management focused on tapering opioid analgesic medications. Opioid analgesic medications were not considered key elements in chronic pain management at the time, and indeed had not been throughout history, because of fears of toxicity, tolerance, and addiction with prolonged use.

Perhaps even more important than the development of multidisciplinary pain clinics was the framing of pain as a biopsychosocial condition. This framing emphasized that advances in treating pain could only come from the study of biology, psychology, and social contributors, requiring the efforts and coordination of many different disciplines. There were already hints that a mechanical model could not capture the full complexity of human pain. As René Leriche is quoted in Bonica's 1953 textbook: "Physical pain is not a simple fact of nervous impulses traveling over a nerve at a predetermined gait. It is the resultant of the conflict between the stimulus and the individual."[3(p145)] The struggle to personalize the mechanical model of pain continues to this day.

Although he had succeeded at fostering pain research in Seattle, Bonica recognized that what was needed to advance the field of pain medicine was an international collaboration of pain clinicians and researchers. In 1973, he invited 350 of the world's leaders in pain treatment and research from 13 different countries to an international forum that took place in a former nunnery in Issaquah, Washington, a suburb of Seattle. Here the idea of an International Association for the Study of Pain (IASP) was raised, leading to its foundation in 1974. The mission of the IASP is to "bring together scientists, clinicians, health-care providers and policymakers to stimulate and support the study of pain and to translate that knowledge into improved pain relief worldwide." Today the IASP has chapters in 96 countries, has fostered multiple other pain societies, and is recognized as the most authoritative voice in the taxonomy, diagnostic coding, messaging, ethics, and politics of pain.

John Bonica was a force of nature who succeeded in achieving an expansive vision for pain study and relief. What he and other early converts in the collaboration between clinicians and scientists could not have predicted was how easy it would be to pervert this vision. Pain relief would become more important than the multidisciplinary approach to understanding and treating human suffering. Lowering the intensity of physical pain would become the primary goal of pain care. This perversion of the pain management ideal is the subject of this book.

Julia Arnold, part 3

Three years later, Julia's abdominal pain has returned. The OB-GYN who operated before again performed laparoscopic surgery. She again found some small areas of endometriosis on the abdominal and bowel wall, which she cauterized. Julia recovered well and thought she had less pain during her menses over the next few months, but after that the pain escalated. It did not respond to your treatment with anti-inflammatories and muscle relaxers. Suppressing Julia's ovulation with birth control pills also did not work. In fact, the pain now extended before and after menstruation to most of the month. The pain had also spread from her abdomen to her back and was limiting her mobility. She was no longer able to work as a hairdresser.

In addition to spreading, Julia's pain seemed to be intensifying. Whereas she had often rated her pain as a 6 on a 10-point scale, she now regularly rated it an 8. She said it interfered with her sleep nearly every night and her mood during the day. She was becoming very discouraged about the possibility of natural improvement of her endometriosis or treatment success for her pain. No one could explain to her why her pain was spreading and intensifying. Another consultation with a new OB-GYN yielded no new ideas about diagnosis or treatment. There did not seem to be any way to remove the endometriosis that was causing Julia's abdominal pain. Yet the pain remained a significant problem for her, disrupting her ability to work and enjoy life.

Cicely Saunders and the parallel growth of palliative care

During Bonica's lifetime, across the Atlantic in Britain, another notable person was breaking ground in the medical care of the dying. Cicely Saunders (Figure 2.2) is credited with founding the palliative care movement, now an established medical discipline. Just as there is a remarkable personal history behind the man who became the renowned John Bonica, so there is a remarkable personal history behind Cicely Saunders. Born in 1918 in Barnet, Hertfordshire, she was admitted to St. Anne's College,

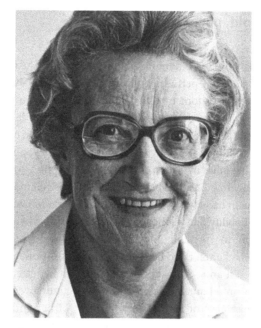

Figure 2.2. Dame Cicely Saunders (1918–2005)
Permission obtained from Derek Bayes Photography

Oxford University, in 1939 to study philosophy, politics, and economics after her father urged her to abandon her long-fostered desire to become a nurse. For a woman at the time, admission to Oxford was already an extraordinary achievement since it was rare for women to be accepted into the highly competitive world of academics. After the outbreak of the Second World War, she defied her father and broke from her studies in Oxford to pursue nursing. She was forced to abandon her nursing career because of back pain. She then switched to social work and became what was then called a "lady almoner," a hospital social worker. While a lady almoner, she was converted to the Christian faith by a group of Christian friends and switched from being agnostic to becoming a devout Christian. She also met and fell in love with a dying 40-year-old Polish man, David Tasma. They developed the idea of a home for dying people to find peace in their final days. In his will, he contributed a substantial sum of money toward a home for dying people, where scientific knowledge could be combined with spiritual comfort.

In 1952, at the age of 33, Saunders was persuaded she would not be taken seriously unless she had a medical degree, so she entered medical school. Once a qualified physician, she took up dual positions as a researcher in pain management for the incurably ill at St. Mary's Hospital, Paddington, and with nuns at St. Joseph's, a hospice for the dying poor in Bayswater, where she used her medical knowledge to guide the nuns caring for the terminally ill. At St. Joseph's she met a second dying Polish man, Antoni Michniewicz, with whom she also had a close spiritual relationship. During this time, and with the help of funding from Tasma, she set in motion the building of the now famous and still existing St. Christopher's Hospice in Hackney, southwest London, which opened in 1967. She herself died of breast cancer in St. Christopher's Hospice in 2005 at the age of 87.

In St. Christopher's Hospice, Cicely Saunders achieved the marriage of spiritual and medical care. Hospices had existed since the mid-1800s, but they were church-based and largely offered spiritual comfort for the "incurable," with no role for medicine. Cicely Saunders believed that the relief of pain by medical means was necessary if dying patients were to engage in the spiritual aspects of preparing for death. She insisted that dying people needed dignity, compassion, and respect, backed by rigorous scientific methodology in the testing of treatments. "Total pain" was the term she used to describe the physical, emotional, social, and spiritual dimensions of distress in dying patients. The way in which her philosophy transformed the care of the dying patient is encapsulated by a quote from a St. Christopher's Hospice patient:

> They used to see how long I could go without an injection. I used to be pouring with sweat because of the pain. I couldn't speak to anyone and I was having crying fits. I think I've only cried once since I've been here ... The biggest difference is feeling so calm. I don't get worked up or upset.[4]

The Brompton Cocktail was a morphine–cocaine elixir prepared with sweet alcohol (the latter largely to reduce the bitter taste of morphine) that was first described by Herbert Snow in 1896 for treating advanced cancer.

It was later taken up for post-thoracotomy pain at the Royal Brompton Hospital in London, after which the elixir was later named. The mixture had become established in Britain for treating pain at the end of life by the time Cicely Saunders opened St. Christopher's Hospice. But she was not satisfied that the cocktail as described by Snow was the best solution for severe pain, and she determined that research was needed in order to advance beyond it.

In 1971, she appointed the 30-year-old Robert Twycross as a clinical research fellow at St. Christopher's Hospice. He was the person who demonstrated that morphine alone (without cocaine) was a better approach for most patients than the cocktail. Throughout the 1970s, he also became a pioneer of the hospice movement with Cicely Saunders, actively building palliative care across the globe. He holds honorary roles in palliative care organizations to this day.

Twycross became aware that Napp Pharmaceuticals, a British company bought by the Sackler brothers from New York in 1966, had developed a new type of extended-release pill known as the Contin delivery system. It combined hydrated cellulose with high aliphatic alcohol to slow down the release of the active drug. The Contin delivery system was first used to make twice-daily aminophylline and theophylline for the treatment of asthma. Twycross believed that a slow-release form of morphine could help his cancer patients, who would not have to take their morphine as often or be woken at night by pain. At the suggestion of Twycross, Napp Pharmaceuticals and Purdue Frederick (now Purdue Pharma), the U.S. company owned by the Sackler brothers, began the development of slow-release morphine. They named their slow-release morphine MS Contin, and it was the first slow-release opioid on the market, launched in 1987. The uses of MS Contin have never extended much beyond the treatment of cancer pain and pain at the end of life. However, using their Contin technology, the Sackler brothers, their descendants, and their company Purdue Pharma went on to develop the blockbuster drug OxyContin, introduced in 1996. OxyContin was developed as MS Contin's patent was running out, to provide the company with alternative newly patented opioid. Turning OxyContin into a medication to treat chronic pain was a ploy to increase sales even further. Purdue and the drug OxyContin have since become household names because of their role in the U.S. opioid epidemic.

A marriage of two visions: pain and palliative care

"Opiophobia"—fear of opioids—is a word coined in the 20th century to make fear of opioids seem irrational. But there is nothing new about fearing opioids; their addictive properties have been known for millennia. Their ability to cause death through respiratory depression grew after the invention of the hypodermic needle in 1844 enabled large doses to reach the brain quickly, and new, more rapidly absorbed opioids, such as heroin, were synthesized in 1874. The devastating effect on populations of widespread use of opioids was already obvious in countries where opium was grown and in plentiful supply. China, for example, had edicts against opium as early as 1729. What was new about 20th-century opiophobia, however, was that for the first time it applied to the treatment of pain with opioids and affected both patients and prescribers. Opiophobia in the clinical pain setting was much more of a problem for the United States than it was for Britain, where the leadership of Cicely Saunders in the care of the dying legitimized opioid use.

Broadly, there are two reasons the United States suffered from opiophobia in the clinical setting more than other developed countries: The first relates to American drug regulations, the second to American cultural attitudes to drug use. The 1914 Harrison Act in the United States and the 1920 Dangerous Drug Act in Britain both made the sale and distribution of opioids and other addictive substances illegal other than for medical purposes. But the two diverged when it came to recreational and medical use. British drug laws (mirrored in other European and Commonwealth countries) were relatively permissive in that they did not punish users, and allowed physicians to treat heroin addiction with heroin or other opioids. The Harrison Act, in conjunction with its subsequent amendment by a 1919 Supreme Court ruling making it illegal to treat opioid addiction with opioids (*Webb v. United States*), restricted the legal use of opioids to medically supervised pain management.

Repressive drug laws in the United States had a chilling effect on physicians, who became reluctant to prescribe opioids even for acute pain, for fear of creating addicts and losing their medical licenses and livelihoods. Attitudes toward intoxication and drug use in the United States, as manifested by Prohibition (1920–1933) and President Richard Nixon's War on Drugs in 1971, are now recognized by many to be excessively punitive and possibly counterproductive.[5] Reflective of American attitudes to drug use are the words of Henry Anslinger, who was commissioner of the Federal Bureau of Narcotics from 1930 to 1962: "Drug addiction is an evil; for it to be rooted out and destroyed, it was only necessary for the USA to behave like 'a well-coached football team, crisp in its blocking, sharp in its tackling and well-drilled in all the fundamentals.'"[6] By 1991, 21% of prison inmates in the United States were incarcerated for drug offenses and the United States already had the highest per capita incarceration rate in the world. These statistics have changed little today.

The hospice movement in the United States was launched in 1974 by a group of students at Yale University inspired by Cicely Saunders's ideals. Home hospice care suited America and its healthcare system better than inpatient hospice. But the principles of inpatient hospice were retained, combining medical control of distressing symptoms with spiritual and family support, with the goal of allowing people to die with dignity and in peace. The hospice movement soon led to the hospital-based palliative care movement of the 1980s, which 10 years later became the fastest growing field in U.S. health care. American medicine's overemphasis on cure had led to an underappreciation of the roles of acceptance, peace, dignity, and pain relief for people with incurable diseases.

What distinguishes palliative care from hospice is the difference between incurable disease and life-limiting disease, and the ability to provide palliation alongside disease-oriented treatments for the former. The challenge for U.S. physicians was not only in overcoming attitudinal barriers to providing palliation, but also overcoming opiophobia, which reached its peak around 1980 just as palliative care was gaining acceptance. Cicely Saunders would not have understood opiophobia, since in Britain, opioids were prescribed at the end of life freely and without fear of censure. But for the pioneers of hospice and palliative care in the United States, much work needed to be done before opioids could be used as freely as they were in Britain.

As the IASP became increasingly involved in global pain initiatives, there arose a marriage between John Bonica's model of chronic pain management and Cicely Saunders's palliative care ideals. But this marriage between these two ideals was to portend disaster for the United States, and for the pain field. That disastrous pairing was the extension of palliative care principles into the management of chronic pain, spearheaded by the palliative care pioneers, who had so successfully improved the care of patients at the end of life. With the best of intentions, they believed that chronic pain would benefit from a similar approach of aggressive control of pain through opioid prescription. However, applying palliative care principles to the treatment of chronic pain was to set up a number of problems, which we discuss throughout this book.

Pain as the fifth vital sign

One of the first priorities for the IASP was to improve pain relief for people dying of cancer. Although the IASP was initially focused on chronic pain, basic science, and research, by the time of its first meeting in Florence in 1975, word of the new society had gotten out into the palliative care world, and a 1-day supplementary symposium on cancer pain followed the First World Congress. The cancer symposium was organized by Vittorio Ventafridda from the National Cancer Institute in Milan and Kathleen Foley from Memorial Sloan Kettering Cancer Center in New York. Interest in the satellite meeting surprised its organizers, and there was standing room only. Among the 150 delegates at the symposium were John Bonica and Robert Twycross, Cicely Saunders's acolyte and the scientific director of her hospice in London. The satellite meeting brought together a group of people who were later to play a key role in the World Health Organization (WHO)'s involvement in promoting cancer pain relief. By the 1980s, the WHO had designated cancer a "major world problem"[7] causing 10% of all deaths, with pain being a major symptom for 70% of people with advanced cancer. At the time (the 1980s), cancer was a rapidly progressive and painful disease that ended in death for most. Cancer pain therefore provided a clear and compelling target for opioid therapy. Draft guidelines for the treatment of cancer pain written by a group of experts brought together in Milan by the WHO in 1982 were finalized at a WHO meeting held in Geneva in December 1984, and released as a book in 1986.[7] Kathleen Foley chaired the 1984 meeting, and both John Bonica and Robert Twycross served on the panel. Experts in cancer pain management were joined by experts in the regulation of opioid drugs, pharmaceutical research and manufacturing, and representatives from several nongovernmental organizations. The goal of the panel was to demystify the use of opioids at the end of life by developing a simple algorithm using common medications, and to promote the implementation of this algorithm by governments and other regulators. The cancer pain experts found that most cancer pain could be successfully controlled with judicious use of opioids arranged on a pathway from mild to strong analgesics. The concept of starting with non-opioid analgesics and graduating through weak opioids to strong opioids as disease and pain progressed was presented as the now widely used WHO "stepladder" approach.

Importantly, the guideline not only promoted the idea of progressing from weak to strong analgesics, but it also specifically recommended dose escalation as needed, stating: "The 'recommended' or 'maximum' doses described in standard textbooks are useful as starting doses only; more is often required. The doses of morphine and other strong opioids can be increased indefinitely."

The WHO's 1986 book *Cancer Pain Relief* introduced three new principles for the prescribing of opioids to treat severe pain: (1) the titrate-to-effect principle, (2) the principle of open-ended dose escalation, and (3) the principle of round-the-clock dosing. These were principles that have helped many cancer patients get effective and safe pain relief, and are still used as a basis for treating pain during progressive painful disease. The WHO cancer pain guideline had been years in the making. During the process, palliative care specialists from the United States were beginning to think that chronic pain was undertreated for similar reasons. Irrational "opiophobia" was diminishing because of successful treatment for cancer patients. Why not apply the same principles for chronic pain patients whose suffering equaled, and sometimes exceeded, that of cancer pain patients?

Also in 1986, Kathleen Foley and her junior colleague Russell Portenoy published a seminal paper: "Chronic use of opioid analgesics in non-malignant pain: Report of 38 cases."[8] In this paper, they describe the successful treatment with opioids of Memorial Sloan Kettering cancer patients for pain unrelated to their cancer. Those patients had very low rates of problematic opioid use (only 2 of the 38) and obtained satisfactory pain relief at moderate opioid doses over a period of years. They concluded that "opioid maintenance therapy can be a safe, salutary and more humane alternative to the options of surgery or no treatment in those patients with intractable non-malignant pain and no history of drug abuse." At the time, there was very little else in the literature to support the use of chronic opioid therapy in patients without cancer. Although it provided a very low level of evidence, Foley and Portenoy's paper was effectively used to promote the idea that opioids could and should be used for the treatment of chronic non-cancer pain.

After the rapid implementation of new principles for treating cancer pain, the slow progress with treating other sorts of pain began to frustrate the pain specialists. Despite their educational efforts and their writing of treatment guidelines, pain was still underrecognized and undertreated, especially in hospitals. To increase its visibility, why not measure and chart it, as had been done in research for some time? In 1996, James Campbell, then president of the American Pain Society (APS), the American chapter of the IASP, introduced the idea of pain as the fifth vital sign, along with the traditional four vital signs of pulse, blood pressure, temperature, and breathing. He stated: "If pain were assessed with the same zeal as other vital signs are, it would have a much better chance of being treated properly."[9]

Julia Arnold, part 4

You have tried every treatment you could think of to help relieve Julia's pain, including anti-inflammatories, muscle relaxers, tricyclic antidepressants, and acetaminophen. She has recently gone to the emergency room for a particularly severe episode of abdominal pain. She received some morphine there that provided significant and immediate relief of her pain. She asks you why you have not prescribed an opioid, since that is the strongest pain medicine. You were reluctant because all the teaching you had received to date cautioned against prescribing opioids for chronic pain because of the risk of addiction. But recently, the teaching had changed, and the pain specialists were beginning to say that the risk of addiction had been overblown, and addiction is very rare when opioids are used as pain treatment. You agree to Julia's request for opioids partly because nothing else seems to have helped, and partly because there is now moral pressure on you to abandon prior caution and prescribe opioids for patients like Julia because refusing to prescribe is tantamount to cruelty. You prescribe Percocet (oxycodone with acetaminophen) 4 times daily as needed, which is 120 tablets for 30 days. After the first 30 days, when Julia's prescription comes up for renewal, she reports her pain level as 4/10, a clear improvement from the 8/10 she reported before opioids were started. She is very happy about this. You are relieved.

In 1998, taking its lead from the APS, the U.S. Veterans Health Administration (VHA), the only government-run healthcare system in the United States, launched a national strategy to improve pain management that required providers to assess and record pain intensity using a 0-to-10 numerical rating scale. Other healthcare systems were much slower to introduce the pain score into clinical practice, but that changed swiftly when in 2001 the body responsible for accrediting U.S. healthcare facilities, the Joint Commission (at the time known as the Joint Commission for the Accreditation of Healthcare Organizations [JCAHO]) mandated standards for the quantitative assessment and management of pain. This initiative was suggested and promoted by pain specialists, frustrated that despite their efforts, pain remained underrecognized and undertreated. Although JCAHO did not specifically require the use of a 0-to-10 pain score, the pain score was very quickly taken up since it was a simple and practical way to comply with the JCAHO pain mandate, and provide the documentation needed to satisfy the scrutiny of the JCAHO quality assessors. The implementation of the JCAHO mandate did not suggest the use of opioids specifically, but a decade later, it is now indisputable that the idea that a high pain score should not be tolerated helped trigger massive increases in opioid prescribing by U.S. doctors. After a steady increase in the overall national opioid dispensing rate from 1999, the total number of prescriptions dispensed in the United States peaked in 2012 at more than 255 million, with a dispensing rate of 81.3 prescriptions per 100 persons, enough for nearly one per adult citizen.[10] Opioids (licit combined with illicit) were involved in 46,802 U.S. overdose deaths in 2018 (70% of all drug overdose deaths).[11] More than 760,000 people have died in the United States since 1999 from a drug overdose.

The role of the pharmaceutical industry

Julia Arnold, part 5

When Julia comes for her third refill of Percocet, she reports that her pain level has climbed back up to 6/10; some days it reaches 8/10. She has been so impressed with the pain relief she has obtained from the Percocet that she asks if she can have a bit more. You have learned from continuing medical education courses that there is no dose of opioids that is the correct dose for everyone. You have been taught that opioids must be titrated to their effect on pain. The right dose is the dose that provides pain relief for the patient. Although you still have some addiction concerns, Julia has not misused her Percocet. You agree to a dose increase. But since the amount of acetaminophen would be too high if you prescribed Percocet, you decide to switch Julia to OxyContin 20 mg twice daily instead. She is happy with this. At her next refill, she reports her pain is back down to 4/10. She has not returned to work, but she is thinking about it.

At this time, few readers will be unaware that the pharmaceutical industry is facing multiple lawsuits concerning the U.S. opioid epidemic. Although the epidemic has now changed into an epidemic of illicit rather than prescription opioid abuse, the case against the industry is that misleading marketing in the 1990s and early 2000s led to an unprecedented increase in prescribing opioids for pain that was responsible for the first wave of the current epidemic. That led to the second wave (an epidemic of heroin abuse and deaths) and the current third wave (an epidemic of fentanyl abuse and deaths). Purdue Pharma, the private company owned by the Sackler brothers, has been the most active in promoting the use of opioids for the treatment of chronic pain. It persuaded prescribers to abandon caution and treat chronic pain with opioids. The Sackler brothers were skilled salesmen, recognized for adapting mass marketing strategies to pharmaceuticals, especially controlled substances.

Arthur, Mortimer, and Raymond Sackler were the sons of immigrants to the United States from Galicia (now Ukraine) and Poland, born in 1913, 1916, and 1920 respectively. They all went to medical school and became psychiatrists. They quickly made a name for themselves as early advocates for medication treatment for psychiatric disorders. Arthur, the oldest brother, became a pioneer in medical advertising and attained fame for philanthropy in the arts. Arthur recognized that medical advertising was a seduction of both prescribers and patients, and he developed marketing techniques to promote benzodiazepines, especially Valium. From 1969 to 1982, Valium was the most prescribed drug in the United States, with sales peaking in 1978 at more than 2.3 billion pills sold. Valium and its marketing strategy were commemorated in the 1966 song by the Rolling Stones, "Mother's Little Helper":

> "Kids are different today"
> I hear ev'ry mother say
> Mother needs something today to calm her down
> And though she's not really ill
> There's a little yellow pill
> She goes running for the shelter of a mother's little helper
> And it helps her on her way, gets her through her busy day

Valium was indeed marketed to doctors as appropriate for mothers who were beset by the stresses of raising toddlers. So adept was Arthur Sackler at medical advertising that in 1997, he was posthumously inducted into the Medical Advertising Hall of Fame. He was praised at the time for "bring(ing) the full power of advertising and promotion to pharmaceutic markets." But the view of Allen Frances, past chair of the Department of Psychiatry at Duke University, was less sanguine: "Most of the questionable practices that propelled the pharmaceutical industry into the scourge it is today can be attributed to Arthur Sackler."[12]

After Arthur Sackler died in 1986, his share of Purdue Frederick passed to his brothers, Mortimer and Raymond. Purdue Frederick moved to its current location in Stamford, Connecticut, and launched MS Contin in 1987. As soon as Arthur's estate could be settled, the company changed its name to Purdue Pharma. The idea was already brewing of developing an extended-release opioid that could be used beyond the cancer pain for which morphine had achieved acceptance. Oxycodone was chosen because it already had acceptability for alleviating pain other than cancer pain, and the development of a second extended-release opioid using Contin technology was accelerated when it was realized in 1990 that MS Contin would soon suffer severe generic competition. OxyContin was released in 1996.

The Sacklers realized that the best way to promote their product was to tap into the evolving beliefs of physicians concerning "customer satisfaction," "taking pain seriously," and even a nascent "right to pain relief," which had begun in palliative care. The Sacklers' technique was to support the voices that were already out there in pursuit of the goals of the company. That is why it is difficult to determine culpability for the opioid epidemic. Were the people to blame those who were trying to improve pain control for the millions of people suffering from uncontrolled pain, or was it the pharmaceutical industry that knew that their marketing was misleading—or should the blame be shared?

Julia Arnold, part 6

Julia has now been on opioid therapy for 10 years. She has gotten some good pain relief, but then this fades over time. You increased the opioid dose, since the teaching now was that poor pain control was probably related to inadequate opioid dose. Julia is now taking 160 mg OxyContin each day. She still had some abdominal pain and some back and neck pain. Nevertheless, she is convinced that the opioids are helping, and she is constantly frightened of having the opioid dose reduced or, worse still, not being able to get hold of opioid treatment if you are no longer her doctor.

It has long been known that opioids are capable of providing comfort in the short term while creating the risk of addiction in the long term, and that makes moral and legal determinations on their use and promotion so difficult. In 1650, Thomas Willis wrote in *Medicine in Man's Body*:

> The Angelic face of Opium is dazzlingly seductive, but if you look on the other side of it, it will appear altogether a Devil. There is so much poison in this All-healing Medicine that we ought not to be by any means secure or confident in the frequent and familiar use of it.[13]

Although Pharma argued that the dangers of opioids had been overstated and that we were suffering from a bad case of opiophobia, history—from the U.S. Civil War to China's Opium Wars—shows that these concerns are well grounded.

Naturally, a drug company wants its products to sell, which means claiming that a product is helping people by improving their health. Most drugs would not be appealing or marketable if they did not achieve their stated outcome. But opioids are different, because opioid dependence means that people will like them and will continue to request them even if they are not achieving their stated goal of safely providing pain relief. This is because withdrawal from opioids is difficult and painful, and may be an insurmountable hurdle for some people. Despite their messaging to the contrary, the Sackler brothers knew that their drug OxyContin was as addictive as any other strong opioid. One might regard their business tactics as unethical because they concealed the addictive properties of OxyContin. When confronted 1 year after the launch of OxyContin with concerns that had arisen in the community concerning its abuse liability, Richard Sackler, the son of Raymond and by then the most active Sackler family member in Purdue Pharma, wrote: "Why don't you guys plan a presentation about addiction.... [You should] give a convincing presentation that [extended-release] products are less prone to addiction potential, abuse or diversion than [immediate-release] products. I think this can be done but defer to BK and RR and other experts."[14]

Years later, in May 2007, Purdue Pharma's president, top lawyer, and former chief medical officer pleaded guilty as individuals to misleading the public about OxyContin's risk of addiction due to its sustained-release properties. They agreed to pay $600 million out of personal funds. In addition, they were charged with a felony and sentenced to 400 hours of community service in drug treatment programs. But the Sacklers escaped personal liability and Purdue went on to earn billions of dollars from OxyContin after that settlement.

Two decades after the heady days in the 1980s when both prescribers and patients had been persuaded that opioid analgesics would be a new dawn for people with pain came the days of reckoning. Prescribed opioids were not as widely or persistently effective as had been hoped, and these opioids had been diverted into the community and caused untold harm. Patients who were hoping for a better life began to struggle with opioid dependence. But who was to blame, and who should pay for the damage? Purdue Pharma and other drug companies had used aggressive marketing tactics to persuade people to use their products—but isn't that expected when running a business? The palliative care specialists who were spokespeople for extending opioids beyond previous usage were passionate believers that people were suffering needlessly because of opiophobia persisting outside the context of cancer pain care. Their goals were surely noble. The professional pain societies representing clinicians and researchers dedicated to finding better ways to manage pain also endorsed more widespread pain assessment and treatment with opioids. The making of pain assessment and treatment into a quality metric was intended to make pain more visible, and ensure that people were not suffering in silence. No doubt all these factors contributed to the vast increase in the prescribing of opioids for pain, leading eventually to the prescription opioid epidemic. But Pharma was able to sell opioids because it was able to exploit preexisting beliefs and values about pain and its treatment. Purdue would have never succeeded in making billions from OxyContin if not for the work of John Bonica, Cicely Saunders, and Kathy Foley as well as the IASP and the Joint Commission.

Julia Arnold, part 7

Julia is now 54 years old. She has now been on opioids for 15 years and is completely disabled by pain. She still takes OxyContin, plus oxycodone for "breakthrough" pain. Her total oxycodone daily dose is 240 mg. You are not so worried about the dose because the latest teaching is that high doses are safe, and the dose needed is whatever dose reduces the pain level. But what does worry you is that the opioid doesn't seem to be working. Julia has not been returned to anything like normal function, as promised when opioids were first promoted as safe and effective for chronic pain in the mid-1990s. In fact, Julia is very depressed, and not improving even though you have tried several antidepressants and benzodiazepines for the treatment of her anxiety. She seems rather out of it, and when you talk to her mother, she tells you that Julia is not the daughter she knows. She sits around all day watching television, has no friends, takes no exercise, and is very short-tempered every time anyone suggests that she is overmedicated, and they are worried about her. The question you now ask (in 2008) is this: Did the opioid help at all, and if not, what else were you supposed to do when nothing else had helped?

Moving from superficial to deep roots of our opioid epidemic

Opioid prescribing in the United States peaked in 2012. Levels had nearly quadrupled since the launch of OxyContin in 1996, bringing parallel increases in lethal opioid overdoses and opioid addiction. The Centers for Disease Control and Prevention has called this "opioid epidemic" a public health crisis. Many remedies for this epidemic have been suggested, but they have generally been inadequate because they are based on superficial analyses of the causes of the epidemic. Professional medicine and medical societies responded with a flurry of continuing medical education courses on the clinical pharmacology of prescribed opioids based on the idea that if physicians knew more about the pharmacokinetics and drug interactions of opioid medications, overdose rates would drop. The U.S. Food and Drug Administration instituted a Risk Evaluation and Mitigation Strategy (REMS) for all long-acting and extended-release opioids.[15] This emphasized patient and prescriber education on using opioids more safely. As a program funded by drug companies, it was based on the flawed idea that it was possible to prescribe opioids more safely without prescribing fewer opioids. Other remedies focused on denying opioids to patients with chronic pain who also had mental health or substance abuse disorders. Various risk stratification schemes were deployed to make sure that opioids were used only for physical pain (pain experienced in the body) and not for other forms of suffering. Despite many varied efforts to focus opioid prescribing on bodily pain, multiple studies show that patients with mental health and substance use disorders are much *more* likely to receive opioids for chronic pain. They also received higher doses for longer periods of time, often with concurrent sedatives.[16,17]

To end our current opioid epidemic and prevent its recurrence, we need to look deeper into its roots, not only at the schemes of greedy pharma entrepreneurs who assured us that opioids were safe, and not only at our misunderstanding of opioids as "painkillers" that leave the rest of the person alone. We need to examine our understanding of pain as a medical problem. We have separated pain from the rest of human suffering as uniquely passive and uniquely "innocent." Our mechanical and medical model of pain sees it as something imposed on the person from outside the boundaries of that person. While other forms of suffering might arise from our beliefs and behaviors, even our identities, this is not our usual view of physical pain. We see this pain as arising from causes outside the person. The person is not responsible for this physical pain and thus can claim a right to be relieved of this pain by medical means. The person with physical pain lacks any agency; he or she is the passive victim of something completely outside their control. Pain is seen to arise from our universal vulnerability to disease, aging, and death, but not from other forms of human suffering. We speak of a right to pain relief, but do not speak of a right to depression relief or a right to anxiety relief. This is because we see pain as a more innocent form of suffering than depression or anxiety. It is an experience imposed on a person from outside the person, even if it arises from inside the body.

In the next chapter, we explore how the new pain medicine and cancer pain movements were combined with the new focus on universal human rights to produce calls for pain relief as a universal human right. In the United States, the Supreme Court played an important role in denying the right to physician-assisted suicide but affirming the right to pain relief through palliative care at the end of life. The general right to pain relief will be an extension of this right not to die in overwhelming pain.

References

1. Osler W. Remarks made on presenting the original papers of W.T.G. Morton to the Royal Society of Medicine on May 15, 1919. *Proc Roy Soc Med*. 1918;65:66.
2. Luhrmann TM. *Of Two Minds: The Growing Disorder in American Psychiatry*. Alfred A. Knopf; 2000.
3. Bonica JJ. *The Management of Pain*. Lea & Febiger; 1953.
4. Richmond C. Dame Cicely Saunders: founder of the modern hospice movement. *Br Med J*. 2005;331:238.
5. Perry MJ. The shocking story behind Richard Nixon's "War on Drugs" that targeted blacks and anti-war activists. American Enterprise Institute. June 14, 2018. www.aei.org/carpe-diem/the-shocking-sickening-story-behind-nixons-war-on-drugs-that-tageted-blacks-and-anti-war-activists
6. Anslinger HJ, Tompkins WF. *The Traffic in Narcotics*. Funk & Wagnalls; 1951:295, 303.
7. World Health Organization. (1986) . Cancer pain relief. World Health Organization. https://apps.who.int/iris/handle/10665/43944

8. Portenoy RK, Foley KM. Chronic use of opioid analgesics in non-malignant pain: report of 38 cases. *Pain*. 1986;25:171–186.

9. American Society of Anesthesiologist Task Force on Pain Management, Acute Pain Section. Practice guidelines for acute pain management in the perioperative setting. *Anesthesiology*. 1995;82:1071–1081.

10. Vital signs: opioid painkiller prescribing. July 2014. Accessed September 29, 2022. https://www.cdc.gov/vitalsigns/opioid-prescribing/index.html

11. U.S. Government. Drug overdose data 2021. Accessed March 18, 2021. https://www.cdc.gov/nchs/pressroom/nchs_press_releases/2022/202205.htm#:~:text=Provisional%20data%20from%20CDC's%20National,93%2C655%20deaths%20estimated%20in%202020

12. Keefe PR. The family that built an empire of pain: the Sackler dynasty's ruthless marketing of painkillers has generated billions of dollars—and millions of addicts. *The New Yorker*, October 23, 2017.

13. Willis T. *Medicine in Man's Body*. Section VI, i, 128. 1650.

14. Chakradhar S, Ross C. The history of OxyContin, told through unsealed Purdue documents. *STAT*. December 3, 2019. https://www.statnews.com/2019/12/03/oxycontin-history-told-through-purdue-pharma-documents/

15. U.S. Food and Drug Administration. Postmarketing requirements for the class-wide extended-release/long-acting opioid analgesics. 2015. https://www.federalregister.gov/documents/2014/04/22/2014-09123/postmarketing-requirements-for-the-class-wide-extended-releaselong-acting-opioid-analgesics-public

16. Seal KH, Shi Y, Cohen G, Maguen S, Krebs EE, Neylan TC. Association of mental health disorders with prescription opioids and high-risk opioid use in US veterans of Iraq and Afghanistan. *JAMA*. 2012;307:940–947.

17. Quinn PD, Hur K, Chang Z, et al. Incident and long-term opioid therapy among patients with psychiatric conditions and medications: a national study of commercial health care claims. *Pain*. 2017;158:140–148.

3
The emergence of a right to pain relief

A change in the meaning of pain

> This bitter fruit of nature hides the seed of a great blessing; it is
> a beneficial effort, a cry of sensitivity through which our intel-
> ligence is warned of the danger menacing us; it is the thunder
> which rumbles before crashing.
>
> A. Hayter, *Opium and the Romantic Imagination*

As discussed in Chapter 2, no single event did more to change attitudes to pain than the birth of anesthesia in 1846. But after centuries of justifying and accepting pain, the idea of abolishing it was not immediately or universally accepted. The Church, the moralists, and even medicine itself found value in pain and feared that its perceived benefits might be spoiled by its relief. The Judeo-Christian tradition saw disease and pain as a punishment from God and eternal life as the reward of suffering pain on Earth. The 19th-century view of pain was that it was normal, a sign of life. A pervasive conviction of physicians at the time was that the presence of pain was necessary for recovery. Some went so far as to suggest that the infliction of pain was therapeutic. There was a belief that pain motivated achievement and artistic creativity—that pain and suffering were prerequisites for genius. Pain could thereby be seen as a supernatural or divine force, the removal of which would blunt accomplishment.[1] The Church and medicine were aligned in their skepticism about the benefits of pain relief. Remarkably, Queen Victoria (1819–1901) changed many minds about the value of pain relief when she proclaimed that anesthesia was acceptable to God. The British monarch, at that time, held huge sway over the culture of the land,

and as head of the Church, she could override the views of the crusty elders of the church: "Dr. Snow gave that blessed chloroform, and the effect was soothing, quieting and delightful beyond measure."[2]

The event that changed American minds on pain and its relief was the Civil War (1861–1865), which followed shortly after the birth of anesthesia. That war's carnage could now be mitigated with a medical response that would both save lives and reduce pain; the humanitarian aspects of anesthesia and pain relief were hard to dispute. As Civil War surgeon Valentine Mott wrote: "I do not believe there is a surgeon of the nineteenth century who would willingly inflict any necessary pain in his operations if once practically acquainted with the means of prevention and once confident and facile in their use."[3] Silas Weir Mitchell, considered the founding father of American neurology and a Civil War physician, described what was probably the first recognized chronic pain condition in the limbs of injured soldiers, for which he coined the name "causalgia." He wrote:

> Perhaps few persons who are not physicians can realize the influence which long-continued and unendurable pain may have upon both body and mind.... Perhaps nothing can better illustrate the extent to which these statements may be true than the cases of burning pain, or as I prefer to term it, causalgia, the most terrible of all the tortures which a nerve wound may inflict.[4(p197)]

Medical care was the path out of pain and the modern hope that we could control the worst aspects of our fate on Earth. It reduced pain from an unconquerable affliction to a potentially soluble problem.

International Association for the Study of Pain becomes the authority on pain

The tools of pain relief expanded rapidly during the second half of the 19th century, and attitudes to pain relief changed with the ability to achieve it. The more tools there were to control pain, the less it seemed necessary to endure pain. By the time John Bonica came on the scene in the 1940s, there was already an acceptance that pain relief could be accomplished, most dramatically through the provision of anesthesia during surgery. Anesthetists by this time were practicing both general and regional anesthesia, the latter by blocking nerves with local anesthetics. The practice of blocking nerves had begun to be extended to the treatment of chronic pain, but it fell to John Bonica to expand the idea of a nerve block clinic into a comprehensive pain management center with wide representation from different disciplines.

Bonica had become increasingly convinced of the need for a team approach for managing complex pain problems during his years as an army physician at Madigan Army Medical Hospital during the Second World War. When he returned to civilian life, he went into practice in Tacoma, Washington, became Chief of Anesthesia at Tacoma General Hospital, and developed the first known multidisciplinary pain clinic. In 1960, Bonica moved to Seattle, where he founded the Department of Anesthesiology at the University of Washington School of Medicine, and, together with Lowell E. White and nurse Dorothy Crowley, established the University of Washington Multidisciplinary Pain Center, which became the seed for the specialty of pain medicine and research, and for the growth of pain clinics around the world.

The 1960s was a time of great growth in the pain field. Not only were pain clinics emerging built on Bonica's model, but there was also renewed interest in the basic science of pain, especially after 1965, when Ronald Melzack and Patrick Wall published the gate control theory of pain,[5] which integrated physiological and psychological concepts. The International Association for the Study of Pain (IASP), which Bonica had founded, held its first meeting as an incorporated body in Florence in 1975. One of the most important achievements of the Florence meeting was the formation of a subcommittee on taxonomy, chaired by Harold Merskey, then of the United Kingdom and later London, Ontario. That committee published its first iteration of pain nomenclature and classification in 1979 in the association's journal *Pain*, which did as much to establish the authority of IASP in matters of pain as did many of its other activities. Not only did the taxonomy become a unifying structure for both pain research and education, but the IASP's definition of pain itself also became widely accepted and promulgated. It is the definition that has helped many people understand the true nature of pain.

Remarkably, the primary text of this definition remained unchanged from 1979 until it was slightly revised in 2020. The 1979 IASP definition of pain is "an unpleasant sensory and emotional experience associated with actual or potential tissue damage, or described in terms of such damage."

Within this definition is an acknowledgment, as Melzack and Wall had established in their gate control theory of pain, that pain is not simply carried in a line-labeled system of neural pathways. Nor is it necessarily an experience caused by sensory input or tissue damage. Because pain is subjective, it exists only as what the person says it is. This definition of pain is based on the groundbreaking work of Harold Merskey in his 1964 thesis *An Investigation of Pain in Psychological Illness*.[6] Merskey maintained his leading role in developing pain terminology throughout many subsequent taxonomy iterations. IASP has continued establishing its authority on matters of pain as, in collaboration with the World Health Organization (WHO), it has played a key role in the development of international pain diagnostic codes (International Classification of Disease [ICD]) that are used by healthcare systems throughout the world concerning the classification of pain conditions. The 2020 definition of pain is changed only in that "described in terms of [damage]" is replaced with "or resembling that associated with [damage]," because "described in terms of" suggests verbal ability which is not needed to experience pain.

John Parr, part 1

John Parr is a 25-year-old male who presented in 1972 to John Bonica's multidisciplinary pain clinic with refractory headaches. In 1968, he was on active duty in Vietnam when he was involved in a roadside explosion and suffered a serious head injury. He was sent back to the United States for treatment and left the military at the end of his term in 1970. His chief pain complaint was intermittent unilateral headache in the temporal and frontal regions occurring 10 to 15 times per week and lasting up to 6 hours per episode, described as severe, throbbing, and piercing. In addition, he complained of constant unilateral neck pain, radiating to the anterior chest. He was not able to work because of the severity and frequency of his headaches. He was taking 30 mg morphine 3 times daily.

Treatment in the pain clinic consisted of weaning him off the opioid over a period of 6 days using a blind methadone taper, a course of cognitive–behavioral therapy, water aerobics, occupational therapy, and drug therapy with carbamazepine and amitriptyline. The opioid wean was entirely in keeping with the thinking of the time, which was that opioids were an impediment to the success of the rehabilitative model of pain care. Four months after receiving rehabilitative therapy in the pain clinic, his headaches were occurring with less frequency and severity, to the extent that he was able to return to the workplace and take up a job as a dispatcher. He also met his future wife during this period.

IASP's relationship with the WHO

IASP's ties with the WHO were not restricted to classifying pain conditions, important though that remains in terms of being able to assess the scale and distribution of pain problems. Another focus for the IASP/WHO partnership was the humanitarian aspect of pain relief. By 1982, the growing relationship between IASP and WHO was sealed at a WHO Consultation Meeting in Pomerio, Italy. Kathleen Foley (Figure 3.1) chaired three expert committees on cancer and palliative care and became a driving force for the

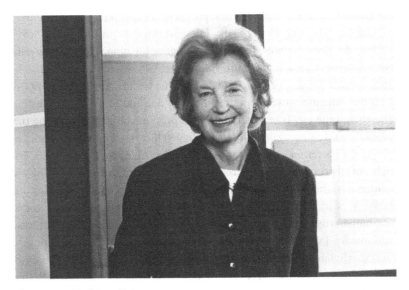

Figure 3.1. Kathleen Foley

From "Neurologist at Work," Memorial Sloan Kettering Cancer Center website, https://www.mskcc.org/experience/physicians-at-work/kathleen-foley-work

groups that developed WHO publications and educational booklets, including *Cancer Pain Relief*. The alliance of IASP, WHO, and palliative care was a major factor in IASP's advocacy for pain relief, and for the use of opioids. This is because undertreatment of pain at the end of life around the world had much to do with unavailability of opioids, or reluctance to use opioids. Before 1982, physicians practicing the new specialty of palliative care felt that end-of-life cancer pain was being undertreated because of unfounded fear of opioids and addiction. In many countries, opioids were not available for dying patients due to local restrictions. But this was to change as principles embodied in the United Nations' Universal Declaration of Human Rights (UDHR, 1948) were extended to include a universal right to the relief of bodily pain.

Evolving concepts of human rights

For at least two centuries, the establishment and extension of human rights has been an important tool and marker of humane progress in the world. After WWII, the abuse and extermination of millions of innocent people on the grounds of race, religion, sexual proclivity, or disability were recognized as "crimes against humanity." Fifty-one governments, including the Soviet Union, the United States, the United Kingdom, China, France, Australia, New Zealand, Canada, and India, joined the UN when it formed in 1945. This number has since grown to include all the world's countries except two with non-member observer status: the Holy See and the State of Palestine. The goal of the UN is to foster peace and prevent conflict by ensuring that people would never again be unjustly denied life, freedom, food, or shelter. The UN Charter was drafted at a meeting in San Francisco in 1945. The rights of all people to freedom from torture and to health and well-being was written into the UN Charter, and ultimately into the UDHR. The idea that everyone worldwide, by virtue of being human, should be entitled to certain human rights had arisen because WWII had witnessed such widespread inhumanity. Previously, people acquired rights by being part of a group—a family, religion, community, class, or state. There had been declarations of human rights in individual countries such as the 1689 English Bill of Rights, the 1789 French Declaration on the Rights of Man and Citizens, and the 1791 U.S. Constitution and Bill of Rights, but many of these declarations excluded sectors of the population such as women and non-whites. The UDHR may have been a turning point in establishing a right of all humans to be spared not only the imposition of pain, but also denial of its treatment. This aspiration for humane treatment was expressed by Emanuel Papper in his 1995 book *Romance, Poetry, and Surgical Sleep*: "Stimulated by the purposes of this book, I began to perceive how pervasive pain and suffering were in the human condition and, paradoxically, how much they were ignored until the ideal of the individual rights of man became acceptable societal perceptions."[1(p24)]

The UN Charter was drafted at a meeting in San Francisco in 1945. The meeting also voted to establish a new international health organization. A year later the WHO Constitution was approved at the International Health Conference in New York. To advance its goal of respecting human rights, the UN established a Commission on Human Rights charged with drafting the UDHR,[7] which was adopted by the UN General Assembly at its third session in Paris on December 10, 1948. The UDHR begins: "Whereas recognition of the inherent dignity and of the equal and inalienable rights of all members of the human family is the foundation of freedom, justice and peace in the world." The UDHR consists of 30 articles affirming individual rights, the 25th of which states: "Everyone has the right to a standard of living adequate for the health and well-being of himself and of his family, including food, clothing, housing and medical care and necessary social services."

Even though the UDHR is not legally binding in any country, countries have invoked it for over half a century, so it has become binding as part of so-called *customary international law*. However, several countries, including the United States, have concluded that the UDHR does not dictate domestic law. Although the Declaration states that people have a "right to medical care adequate for the health of self and family," the United States is one of few countries that signed on to the original UDHR that to this day does not provide universal healthcare.

Even though the whole ethos of the UN was centered on the rights of all humans to be relieved of unjustly imposed suffering or inadequate provision for the relief of suffering, it took several decades for the principles embodied in the UDHR to be extended to an explicit statement regarding a universal right to the relief of bodily pain. General Comment No. 14 was not added until the year 2000: "attention and care for chronically and terminally ill persons, sparing them avoidable pain and enabling them to die with dignity."[8]

Part of this delay was due to the natural fear that a right to pain relief would be seen as a right to opioids.

The UN and the WHO needed to balance the fear that widespread availability of opioids would increase abuse against its humanitarian goal to relieve suffering. The 1961 UN Single Convention of Narcotic Drugs, which set out to develop quotas for medical opioid needs by nation, declared that medical use of opioid medication was indispensable for the relief of pain, and mandated adequate provision of opioids for medical purposes. In 1961, the quotas were calculated based on opioid need for the treatment of cancer and acute pain, which were the only indications for which opioids were considered necessary at the time. But physicians practicing the new specialty of palliative care still felt that end-of-life cancer pain was being woefully undertreated because of unfounded fear of opioids and addiction, often reflected in local restrictions on opioid availability.

Palliative care as a human right

It was through palliative care that the right to pain relief became equated with the right to life itself. As stated by Kathleen Foley: "Providing [pain] relief is vital not only as an end in itself but also to improve the patient's prospects for survival. Pain can erode a patient's willingness to continue treatment, even to live." Foley went on to become a leading opponent of physician-assisted suicide, arguing that palliative treatment could restore dignity and the will to live, and was preferable to suicide and euthanasia:

> Palliative care affirms life, and regards dying as a normal process; neither hastens nor postpones death; provides relief from pain and other distressing symptoms; integrates the psychological and spiritual aspects of patient care; offers a support system to help patients live as actively as possible until death; and offers a support system to help the family cope during the patient's illness and their own bereavement.[9]

The palliative care movement, led by dedicated physicians like Foley, has continued to grow since the pioneering days of Cicely Saunders and Robert Twycross. This movement has helped focus care on the dying person, as medicine has become more focused on the technical aspects of controlling disease and death and has often lost touch with the person who is suffering.

Although the palliative care movement and IASP have tended to diverge over the years, there was considerable overlap in the early days. To this day it is impossible to sever the ties between IASP's focus on pain relief from palliative care's focus on symptom relief during intractable illness. In 1978, 3 years after the IASP satellite meeting in Florence that had brought together leaders in cancer pain management, another landmark meeting, organized by Vittorio Ventafridda, took place in a convent on one of the Venetian islands. The meeting was a combined meeting of the U.S. National Cancer Institute, the National Cancer Institute in Milan, and St. Christopher's Hospice in London. It was the first International Symposium on Cancer Pain, and out of the meeting came a massive tome on cancer pain relief edited by Bonica and Ventafridda: *Advances in Pain Research and Therapy*.[10]

At the meeting, Twycross famously argued with Raymond Houde (a physician expert in analgesics from Memorial Sloan Kettering Cancer Center [MSKCC] in New York, and mentor to Kathleen Foley) about opioid analgesic tolerance. The debate concerned what dosing regimen is needed, considering whether tolerance to opioids' analgesic effects exists. Their argument was reflected in WHO's *Cancer Pain Relief* and led to the establishment of the titrate-to-effect principle, which became important as opioids began to be used for chronic pain.

Cardinal Albino Luciani of Venice, who later became Pope John Paul I, met with delegates of the 1978 Venice meeting. The interest that the Catholic Church had in the dual efforts of the hospice movement and the IASP continued in 1987 when IASP member Corrado Manni from the Universita Cattolica del Sacro Cuore in Rome arranged for a private audience with Pope John Paul II to present the work of IASP. The private audience took place in the Pope's glorious summer residence in Castel Gandalfo, immediately preceding IASP's Fifth World Congress in Hamburg, Germany. Incoming IASP president Michael Cousins, as well as Ronald Melzack, Louisa Jones, John Bonica, and their families, were part of the private audience. For the Catholics among them, the audience with the Pope was a highlight in their lives, never to be forgotten. IASP is a secular organization, but the humanitarian aspect of its work has often attracted leaders with deep religious and spiritual motivations. These pain leaders have always seen themselves as on a moral mission to relieve suffering.

The maturing of palliative care as a medical discipline coincided with growing global health initiatives that began after WWII. These initiatives aimed to reduce human disease and suffering through several covenants written to establish the principles of individual dignity, universality, and nondiscrimination. The International Bill of Rights (1948) comprises three documents drafted under the auspices of the UN: the UDHR, the International Covenant on Civil and Political Rights (ICCPR), and the International Covenant on Economic, Social and Cultural Rights (ICESCR). General Comment No. 14, written by the ICESCR committee,[8,11] specifically attests that all persons, regardless of social status or medical condition, have a right to palliation and relief of pain.

Despite these assertions, there were still many barriers to the implementation of palliative care in healthcare systems, including political, ethical, and regulatory barriers to the availability of opioids. For example, it was much easier to find acceptance of palliative care principles in the United Kingdom than in the United States. In Cicely Saunders's time, U.K. patients accepted their physicians' paternalistic determination that it was time for comfort measures. The American character was much more in line with fighting to the bitter end, and U.S. laws were ambiguous regarding the legality of possibly hastening death. Was it permissible to use opioids to relieve a patient's pain (a legitimate act) when doing so might shorten the patient's life through sedation and respiratory depression (an illegitimate effect)? This dilemma is embodied in the *principle of double effect*, a set of ethical criteria that Christian philosophers and others have proposed for evaluating the permissibility of carrying out a legitimate act that might result in a bad outcome. The act itself must be good or at least morally neutral, the intent of the act must be good, and there must be sufficient justification for the good, even if the actor knows of possible harm or evil. The principle of double effect has been applied to relief of suffering at the end of life, when the palliative treatment could inadvertently hasten death, or be seen as assisting suicide.

The principle of double effect relies on the distinction between intended and unintended effects of an action taken to relieve suffering. In the clinical care of dying patients, this difference can be difficult to discern. In 1997, the U.S. Supreme Court agreed to hear two cases that posed two questions related to the issue of hastening death in terminally ill patients: (1) Is there a constitutional right to assistance in suicide? (2) Is the right to refuse life-saving treatment the same as a right to receive assistance in committing suicide? The first question was addressed in the appeal of the Ninth Circuit Court's opinion on Washington's law (*Washington v. Glucksberg*), and the second in the appeal of the Second Circuit Court's opinion on New York's law (*Vacco v. Quill*).[8] Although the court denied the right to assisted suicide in each case, the court was very clear that palliative care with the primary intention of relieving pain and suffering, and with the patient's consent, should be strongly encouraged. At least five members of the court emphasized the "right not to suffer," at least when death is imminent, which was seen as a warning to the states not to prohibit physicians from doing everything in their power to relieve pain and suffering at the end of life.

The Supreme Court thus unanimously ruled that there was no constitutional right to assisted suicide but asserted an alternative right to palliative care. As Robert Burt summarized in the *New England Journal of Medicine*:

> A Court majority effectively required all states to ensure that their laws do not obstruct the provision of adequate palliative care, especially for the alleviation of pain and other physical symptoms of people facing death. (affirming this right, even if it hastened death).[12(p1234)]

Justice Sandra Day O'Connor specifically made this point:

> A patient who is suffering from a terminal illness and who is experiencing great pain has no legal barriers to obtaining medication, from qualified physicians, even to the point of causing unconsciousness and hastening death.[13(p1527)]

Writing in the *Journal of the American Medical Association*, Lawrence Gostin concluded:

> More importantly, the Court's decision could be read for proposition that the state could not, consistent with the Constitution, prosecute a physician for causing a patient's death, where that death was a secondary consequence of aggressive pain management.[13(p1528)]

Here pain relief was recognized as an adequate reason for a patient to die if the death was not explicitly intended. This is a very strong endorsement of the right to pain relief. However, the Court addressed the right to pain relief only in the context of palliative care for the dying.

The international push for the rights of people to receive palliative care was also gaining momentum. Although that right was already articulated in the International Bill of Rights, by the 1990s there was broad recognition that it was not enough: People across the globe were suffering unnecessarily for lack of palliative care services. Several countries instituted their own claims that end-of-life care was the right of every citizen. The international palliative care community issued a number of key statements, including the Cape Town Declaration (2002),[14] the Korea Declaration (2005),[15] and the Budapest Commitments (2007),[16] which called for governments to:

1. Create and implement palliative care policies
2. Provide services equitably, without discrimination
3. Make available critical medications, including opioids
4. Provide palliative care at all levels of care
5. Integrate palliative care education at all levels of learning and for all caregivers

What became known as the Budapest Commitments comprised the European Association of Palliative Care (EAPC), the International Association of Hospice and Palliative Care (IAHPC), and the Worldwide Palliative Care Alliance (WPCA). In collaboration with Human Rights Watch and IASP, the international palliative care community argued for the end of discrimination against patients in pain and dying and the lifting of "draconian" domestic opioid laws, policies, and practices that restrict opioid availability, accessibility, and affordability.[11] In conjunction with World Palliative Care Day in 2008, the IAHPC and WPCA published its Joint Declaration and Statement of Commitment on Palliative Care and Pain Treatment as a Human Right.[17] IASP designated 2008–2009 its Global Year Against Cancer Pain. Sustained advocacy by the IAHPC and WPCA persuaded two UN Special Rapporteurs on the Right to Health and on Torture to make a clear statement about pain management and palliative care as human rights:

The failure to ensure access to controlled medicine for the relief of pain and suffering threatens fundamental rights to health and to protection against cruel inhuman and degrading treatment. International human rights law requires that governments must provide essential medicine which include, among others, opioid analgesics as part of their minimum core obligations under the right to health. Lack of access to essential medicine, including for pain relief, is a global human rights issue and must be addressed forcefully.[18]

To this day, pain at the end of life is often woefully undertreated, especially in developing nations. The global advocacy for making opioids more available for this indication continues. But unfortunately, the opioid epidemic in the United States, with its acceleration of premature deaths by overdose, has made the case for opioid liberalization in other countries much harder to make.

No treatise on the right to pain relief would be complete without acknowledging the significant role played by Kathleen Foley in advancing palliative care in the United States and around the globe. She came to pain medicine by accident. In 1974, when she was completing her training in neurology at MSKCC, she was offered a research fellowship to study pain. She wanted to do research but had not considered pain. Once she learned how inadequate pain treatment was for cancer patients, she never looked back. Her organization, with Vittorio Ventafridda, of an international symposium on cancer pain in Florence in 1975 began her relationship with IASP, WHO, and the global palliative care community. In 1981, under her leadership, MSKCC opened the first designated pain center in a cancer hospital in the United States. Her advocacy and leadership have been tireless and continue to the time of writing. She was at the forefront of the movement against physician-assisted suicide and co-edited the book *The Case Against Suicide: For the Right of End-of-Life Care*, in which she argued that better end-of-life care would avert the desire to die. Not only did she direct research and clinical programs at MSKCC, but she has also had leadership roles in many national and international palliative care and pain organizations. She has written numerous papers and books and is the recipient of many awards, including the John D. Loeser Distinguished Lecture Award from IASP, of which she is an honorary member. In 2017, she was selected by Pope Francis to a multidenominational Bioethics Advisory Board—a mark of her importance in human protections.

The right to pain relief, the right to opioids: a tangled web

The 1997 Supreme Court ruling was one of several factors that helped remove the shackles of "opiophobia" in the United States in the 1990s. Even though the court had specified "at the end of life," its ruling changed attitudes to opioids not just for those terminally ill, but also for those suffering from chronic pain. Other efforts were under way at the same time to remove barriers to opioid prescribing. The American Pain Society and the American Academy of Pain Medicine wrote a joint statement endorsing the use of opioids in the treatment of chronic pain in 1996, published in 1997.[19] This was followed in 1998 by the Model Guidelines for the Use of Controlled Substances, which was a policy statement of the Federation of State Medical Boards of the United States. In response, at least 20 states passed new laws, regulations, or policies liberalizing the prescribing of opioids when treating pain.[20] These "intractable pain acts" removed limits on the dose and duration of opioid therapy that had been a part of state laws for decades, and contained statements such as "No disciplinary action will be taken against a practitioner based solely on the quantity and/or frequency of opioids prescribed"

In this 21st century, every country has strict laws and regulations that control the production, importation, distribution, and sales of pharmaceutical opioids, and the International Narcotics Control Board (an independent body linked to the UN) imposes similar controls on global access. These tight controls exist not because opioid medications have side effects, including death—many less controlled pharmaceutical products have that potential, even those available over the counter—but because opioid medications are addictive. Societies control the availability of addictive substances not so much to protect individuals, but to protect society itself. Before international trading made opium widely available in Western nations (opium production being in hot climates), controls on opioid use per se were not deemed necessary in the West. But in the East and Middle East, where the opium poppy (for a long time the only source of opioids) was grown, widespread use worried the authorities, and dictums against opioids were introduced centuries before such dictums spread globally. In China, a 1799 imperial proclamation prohibited the cultivation of poppies and the importation or use of opium altogether:

The Celestial Empire does not forbid you people to make and eat opium, and diffuse the custom in your native place. But that opium should flow into the interior of this country, where vagabonds clandestinely purchase and eat it, and continually become sunk into the most stupid and be-sotted state … is an injury to the manners and minds of men.[21(p43)]

The British, who had begun cultivating opium poppies in India, noticed the devastating effects that widespread opium use could have on a society:

If something of this kind is not done, and done quickly too, the thou-sands that are about to emigrate from the plains into Assam will soon be infected with the Opium-mania—that dreadful plague which has depop-ulated this beautiful country, turned it into a land of wild beasts, with which it is overrun, and has degenerated the Assamese from a fine race of people to the most abject, servile, crafty and demoralized race in India.[22]

The first U.S. controlled substances act, the 1914 Harrison Act, was intro-duced because addiction in the United States resulting from domestic treat-ment of everyday pain with opium and morphine elixir (laudanum) began to concern the authorities. But far from controlling use or production, both increased exponentially over the ensuing century.

The importance of this history is that it helps our understanding of atti-tudes and beliefs about opioids that seem indelible and continue to haunt the debate about pain relief. That widespread, uncontrolled opioid use damages societies is not in dispute. Opioid addiction and dependence have reliably emerged in the wake of widespread opioid use. Addiction has long been rec-ognized as a risk of opioid use, whether as a moral failing in the traditional understanding or as a brain disease in the modern formulation. Pain relief, on the other hand, is seen as good, humane, worthy, and necessary. The very roots of palliative care lay in the hospice idea, where dying people could find comfort from good and dedicated people who, after Cicely Saunders's ex-ample, saw the necessity to provide medical relief of pain in conjunction with spiritual care. People who provide pain relief are usually seen as good; people who deny pain relief are often seen as hateful zealots.

Fear of opioids had become very deeply rooted by the mid-20th century, especially in the United States, which had particularly draconian drug laws. Although there is no reason to believe that dying in agony because of lack of availability of opioids was anything new, what hospice and palliative care movements did was to draw attention to the fact that it did not need to be that way. Palliative care offered a better way to die and should be considered part of people's newly established right to humane treatment. In the Cicely Saunders tradition, palliative care attended to "total pain," encompassing bodily, emotional, social, and spiritual pain and suffering. But she believed that medically achieved pain reduction was essential to achieving total pain relief, and opioids were essential for medically achieved pain reduction. She also believed in the importance of scientific validation. As the palliative care field grew, scientific evidence (i.e., trials) confirmed that opioids were an invaluable and irreplaceable tool during end-of-life care. It was also clear that addiction arose rarely, if at all, when opioids were used to treat pain at the end of life. Despite huge hurdles, the palliative care movement was successful in improving pain care for many at the end of life. It also demonstrated that opioids were a safe and effective tool in this effort. Trouble for the pain field lay ahead, not because its intentions were bad, but because its calculations about opioid dependence and addiction were wrong.

Pain relief as a human right

The Memorial Sloan Kettering Cancer Center generally admits only patients with cancer to its services, but it provides comprehensive and long-term care for its patients. Pain is not something that necessarily goes away when cancer is in remission, and the pain that patients with cancer experience is not necessarily related to their cancer. Pain is ubiquitous, and a patient with cancer can suffer nonstructural low back pain as easily as anybody. Very quickly after the formation of the pain clinic at MSKCC in 1981, the providers recognized that the pain they were treating had sometimes evolved into what was called at the time "non-malignant" pain. The distinction between cancer versus non-cancer or non-malignant pain was easier to make in 1981 than it is now because cancer today is rarely a rapidly fatal disease. The MSKCC providers who had been instrumental in persuading political and medical communities of opioids' efficacy and safety at the end of life began to be convinced that opioids could also be used safely for long-term pain relief and non-cancer diagnoses. Very few of their patients (less than 5%) ran into problems taking opioids, and most seemed satisfied with the treatment and reported good pain relief. There had been previous small studies in the early 1980s reporting success with chronic opioid treatment, but none had the impact of Russell Portenoy and Kathleen Foley's aforementioned 1986 study "Chronic Use of Opioid Analgesics in Non-Malignant Pain: Report of 38 Cases."[23] Whether because of the high profile of the authors or their tirelessness in promoting their beliefs, this single case series became a linchpin for the movement that followed—a movement to change people's minds about the suitability and safety of opioid treatment of chronic pain. They were convinced that addiction rates would be low. At the same time, they recognized

> that the efficacy of this therapy and its successful management may relate as much to the quality of the personal relationship between physician and patient as to the characteristics of the patient, drug, or dosing regimen. This is an alternative hypothesis for the positive results reported in this and other studies which has not been directly addressed. The likelihood that the intensive involvement of a single physician does impact favorably on the outcome of opioid maintenance therapy suggests that guidelines for management should include this element.

Now everything was aligned for the pain field to start embracing the idea that caution about chronic opioid therapy had been wrong. The experience of some prominent members of the pain field had been that addiction was a rare occurrence if opioids were given to counteract severe pain. They had no data to support this position in the case of long-term usage. One might ask why the U.S. Food and Drug Administration (FDA) approved these medications for chronic pain. The FDA argued that its role was to assess efficacy and safety on the basis of randomized controlled trials. These trials did demonstrate efficacy and safety for chronic pain, but only for weeks.

Bear in mind that the field of pain management had existed for nearly 20 years. The membership of IASP, scientists and clinicians on a quest to improve people's pain worldwide, had swelled from 975 to 2500 (today it is over 7900). There had been enormous scientific advances in the understanding of pain, addiction, psychology, and opioids. Yet chronic pain and pain disability rates were rising, not falling. Advocacy for the right of people to receive opioids at the end of life was well under way, and pain and palliative care fields were beginning to argue that chronic pain caused equal suffering. Passions were high, and the time was ripe for advancing the candidacy of opioids as a means of reversing the unpalatable trends. After all, if opioids can be used without risk of addiction for 95% of those treated, why should that 95% suffer needlessly?

When, in 1990, Ronald Melzack wrote "The Tragedy of Needless Pain," he was one of the most respected people in the pain field. He had been a founding member and was a past president of IASP. Together with another founding member, Patrick Wall, he had proposed the game-changing "gate control" theory of pain, which turned pain science on its head because it introduced the idea that pain could be modulated. He developed the famous McGill Pain Questionnaire, which is used to this day in both original and modified forms, use of which brought attention to the multidimensional nature of pain. When Melzack spoke, people listened. His 1990 article[24] was published in *Scientific American* under the banner headline:

The Tragedy of Needless Pain
Contrary to popular belief, the author says, morphine taken solely to control pain is not addictive. Yet patients worldwide continue to be undertreated and to suffer unnecessary agony

What Melzack wrote was:

Sadly there are some kinds of pain that existing treatments cannot ease. That care givers can do little in these cases is terribly distressing for everyone involved but is certainly understandable. What seems less understandable is that many people suffer not because their discomfort is untreatable but because physicians are often reluctant to prescribe morphine. Morphine is the safest, most effective analgesic (painkiller) known for constant, severe pain, but is also addictive for some people. Consequently, it is typically meted out sparingly, if it is given at all.

Many care givers, afraid of turning patients into addicts, deliver amounts that are too small or spaced too widely to control pain. Yet the fact is that when patients take morphine to combat pain, it is rare to see addiction.[24(p27)]

Melzack went on to cite the sentinel 1986 Portenoy and Foley 38-patient case series report and its low addiction rates. He also later stated that "patients who develop rapid and marked tolerance to, and dependence on, the narcotics are usually those who already have a history of psychological disturbance or substance abuse." Melzack is quoted here not to be critical of the man now that the benefit of hindsight reveals some errors in his thinking, but because he was a powerful voice, and his words echo what many people in the pain field were thinking and saying at the time.

John Parr, part 2

John Parr presented again to the pain clinic in 1995 at the age of 48 years, after a hiatus of 23 years. His primary care physician felt he had reached the end of the road and did not know how to help. John had experienced several "good" years during which his headaches occurred infrequently; were controlled by non-opioid medication, exercise, bed rest, relaxation, and occasional days off work; and did not interfere too much with his life. He had married, and the couple had 2 daughters. But over time his headaches worsened; his neck pain also worsened and became increasingly disabling. Because he was unable to continue to carry out the physically challenging job of dispatcher, he was reassigned to a desk job.

Ten years after John's first experience in the pain clinic, his primary care physician was persuaded to try an opioid again. Opioid treatment of chronic pain was now encouraged rather than discouraged. In fact, it was now thought unethical to withhold opioids. John was prescribed Percocet (oxycodone/acetaminophen) every 4 hours as needed for the treatment of severe headache. The opioid helped enormously, he became less fearful of his headaches because he knew they would respond to the opioid, and his functional impairment due to neck and arm pain improved. Unfortunately, however, his dose requirement had increased to a level that frightened the primary care physician, and John's absenteeism had resulted in the loss of his job. Accordingly, the primary care physician sought help from the pain clinic. The recommendation of the pain clinic was that John start a long-acting opioid at equivalent dosage, and that he apply for disability.

The journey toward declaring not just palliative care, but pain relief itself, a basic human right occurred under the leadership of another pioneer
in the pain field, Michael Cousins (Figure 3.2). Cousins was a master per-
suader. He represented the pain field in Australia over the entire span of
his very long career, and probably had more influence on how pain was
managed there than any other single individual. As a young anesthetist in
Sydney in the late 1960s, he undertook a postgraduate fellowship in acute
pain management and worked for a while in McGill University, Montreal,
which was pioneering the use of epidural pain relief. Between 1970 and
1974 he worked at Stanford University, California. During his time living
and working in Canada and the United States, he interacted with Ronald
Melzack, Patrick Wall, and John Bonica, which vastly broadened his
horizons.

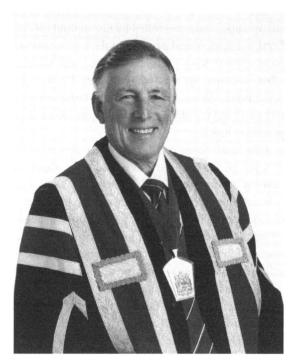

Figure 3.2. Michael Cousins (1939–)
With permission from the Geoffrey Kaye Museum of Anaesthetic History, Melbourne,
Australia

Cousins went back to Australia determined to build pain services and research in Australia much as Bonica was doing in the United States. He thus became part of the grand global scheme to improve pain management. His first task was to develop a multidisciplinary pain center at Flinders Medical Center in Adelaide, after which he moved back home to Sydney and developed another large multidisciplinary pain center at the Royal North Shore Hospital. Both centers became internationally recognized in their time. In 1979 he became the founding president of the Australian Pain Society, and in 1987 he became president of IASP. He played a key role in the formation of an official relationship between IASP and WHO. He raised funds for pain research and education through the nonprofit community-based organization Pain Management Research Institute Ltd., which he founded in the 1990s. In 1995, he was made a Member of the Order of Australia for "service to medicine particularly in the fields of pain management and anesthesia." By 1999 he had become the Founding Dean of the Faculty of Pain Medicine, and in 2005 he played a key role in the recognition by the Australian government of pain medicine as an independent medical specialty.

Influenced by his role in IASP, his palliative care colleagues, and his perception that acute pain management could be better, Cousins long held the view that pain relief, not just palliative care, should be considered a fundamental human right. He had been thinking and writing about the humanitarian aspects of pain relief since the 1980s. In his 1999 Rovenstine Memorial Lecture,[25(p541)] he wrote:

In 1948, the United Nations Declaration of Human Rights said that "all persons are equal in dignity and rights and have the right to life, liberty and security." One can obtain that document incidentally on the Internet, and you will find that it is implied that, with appropriate medical care, one is able to achieve the aim of some quality of life. Interestingly, the United Nations Declaration does not mention pain relief as being a human right. However, I ask you just to ponder what would be your priority list for basic human rights. Would you consider freedom from hunger, which has been discussed so extensively? Freedom from thirst? Peace without political or other persecution? Freedom of speech, press, religion, assembly, mobility? Certainly, these are all important. However, they are difficult to enjoy if one has unrelenting, severe pain. I put it to you that the relief of severe, unrelenting pain would come at the top of a list of basic human rights.

In the year 2000, he wrote in the *Medical Journal of Australia*, "Relief of acute, severe pain is a basic human right, limited only by our ability to provide it safely in the circumstances of individual patients."[26(p3)]

Frank Brennan and Daniel Carr were natural allies in Cousins's quest to establish pain relief as a basic human right. Brennan was a palliative care physician/lawyer in Sydney who had published widely about the human rights dimensions of palliative care. Carr was an endocrinologist, anesthesiologist, and advocate leading the movement to embrace evidence-based acute pain management in the United States. The year 2004 was a banner year for their efforts. A "Global Day Against Pain" was launched by the WHO, in partnership with the IASP and the European Federation of IASP Chapters (EFIC). The theme of the global day was "Pain Relief: A Universal Human Right." In an editorial with the same title published in the IASP's journal *Pain*,[27(p2)] Cousins, Brennan, and Carr wrote:

> Failure to provide relief when this is available is a form of abandonment. In extreme cases it could be regarded as "torture by omission." . . . The bioethical principle of justice can be used to assess the massive humanitarian and financial costs of severe pain and to argue to pain relief as a high social priority. A virtue ethics approach also places pain as a high priority. The current lack of a strong application of these principles to pain relief raises questions about the ethical foundations of current healthcare.

In time, Cousins went on to spearhead an initiative at IASP to write a declaration that the provision of pain treatment should be considered a fundamental human right. In 2010, he chaired the steering committee that developed an International Pain Summit in conjunction with the 13th World Congress in Pain held in Montreal. The "Declaration of Montreal: Declaration That Pain Management Is a Fundamental Human Right" was drafted during this summit; it was later approved by the IASP Council and published in 2011.

But by 2010, there was already a backlash against Cousins, Brennan, and Carr's idea that access to opioids for the treatment of chronic pain was part of the fundamental human right to pain relief. In their 2004 article, they did not specifically call out opioids, but in 2007, when they wrote another more comprehensive article, "Pain Management: A Fundamental Human Right,"[28] they did. In fact, they cited several initiatives in the United States to liberalize opioids for the treatment of chronic pain and called for liberalization of national policies on opioid availability. They suffered a backlash from others in the field who worried that their arguments were purely philosophical and not evidence-based, and that their framing of a right to opioids would result in opioid overprescribing.[29] By 2007, alarming data on rises in prescription opioid abuse admissions and death rates were coming out of the United States,[30] and by the time the framers of the Declaration of Montreal met in 2010, there was caution in the room about promoting opioids: The document itself was careful to promote neither access to pain "relief" nor opioids, but instead access to *pain management*. To pain specialists, "pain management" meant multidisciplinary pain care. But it did not mean much to primary care providers, who knew few pain management techniques beyond opioids.

Nobody could accuse Kathleen Foley, Michael Cousins, Frank Brennan, or Daniel Carr of having any other than the highest motives for promoting opioid therapy for the treatment of distressing pain. They had humanitarian goals, they dedicated their lives to those humanitarian goals, and they labored under the belief of the time that when opioids were used for serious pain, they would rarely be addictive. But that belief was based on the experience that opioids used at the end of life or in hospital settings for short-lived pain are rarely, if ever, addictive. This belief was reinforced by the low rates of addiction in studies such as the seminal 1986 study by Portenoy and Foley, which had been conducted by careful physicians in a controlled setting treating a subset of patients not generalizable to the general population.

But unfortunately, those favorable experiences did not extend to the wider population. As Portenoy and Foley said themselves, "the efficacy of this therapy and its successful management may relate as much to the quality of the personal relationship between physician and patient as to the characteristics of the patient, drug, or dosing regimen."[23(p180)] That proved to be a key element in what followed. Prescribers and patients alike began to struggle with what, other than a high pain score, was the right indication for opioids. Treating those with the highest pain scores selected patients with significant mental health and substance abuse comorbidities (who had been excluded from the randomized trials of opioids for chronic pain) for opioid treatment. Clinical experience went on to reveal that the opioid treatment did not help over the long term, and addiction rates were much higher than had been predicted.

America's opioid epidemic

In no country other than the United States have prescription opioid misuse, abuse, and death rates reached epidemic proportions. These problems increased in parallel with increased prescribing for chronic pain. More and more pain conditions were being treated with opioids using higher and higher doses. Prescription opioid misuse was called out as an epidemic in 2012, but this was only the first wave of the current opioid epidemic in the United States (Figure 3.3). The prescription opioid epidemic evolved into a heroin epidemic and then into the even more lethal fentanyl epidemic. But all these epidemics originated with the widespread prescription of opioids for pain.

A disastrous combination of a push by the pharmaceutical industry and by the pain field to utilize opioids for the treatment of pain, and then an influx of heroin from Mexico and of illicit fentanyl from China, led to today's epidemic. All epidemics are related to access, availability, and exposure. For prescription opioids, the problem was a sudden increase in prescribing that pain specialists interpreted as a correction to the undertreatment of pain, but

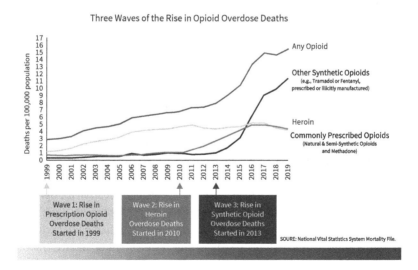

Figure 3.3. The three waves of the opioid epidemic

From Centers for Disease Control and Prevention: Understanding the Opioid Overdose Epidemic, https://www.cdc.gov/opioids/basics/epidemic.html

in fact led to excess prescription drug quietly seeping into the community. For the first time, drug traffickers were not responsible for a drug abuse epidemic: Users themselves were diverting the supplies, which were difficult to distinguish from legitimately prescribed opioids.[31,32] There have been many interventions in the United States to try and encourage more rational use of opioids when treating pain, and to monitor misuse and unsanctioned prescribing. These interventions have stopped the most egregious abuses like "pill mills," but they have not ended the epidemic. The moral tug of war between the right to pain relief and the need to protect patients and the public from opioids continues to this day. Prescribing rates for opioids have gone down in the United States, and abuse and death rates directly related to prescription opioids have also declined. But even after years of effort to control the epidemic, the United States still consumes 75% of the world's prescription opioids for 5% of the world's population. Opioid prescribing in 2020 was still more than twice what it had been in 1999.

John Parr, part 3

By the time John was in his 60s, he was seriously disabled by pain. His wife had left him, and his daughters had become independent adults. He was socially isolated and spent most of his days watching television. He saw his daughters occasionally but did not have any friends. His only trips outside the home were to the shops for necessities, and for occasional walks around the block. He did not feel competent or well enough to own a dog. His only medication was oxycodone at a very high dosage (860 mg per day), which he reported as being the only medication that helped his headaches. He had given up on all other medications.

By this time (2015), the medical community had recognized the dangers of high-dose opioids and was beginning to write new recommendations that suggested dose limits for chronic opioid therapy, and much more restrictive criteria for starting people on opioids. But for John, coming off opioids, or reducing the dose, would not be an easy task. Again, the pain clinic was enlisted to help. This meant that John now received a thorough evaluation of his past traumas and present stresses, including significant events during his childhood, his tour of Vietnam, and his marriage breakup. Treatment now included psychotherapy and psychopharmacology. John, like many other people who have been receiving high doses of opioid for a long time, found tapering very difficult. But with patience, and a determination to improve on his part, his opioid dose decreased, and his state of mind improved. He began to rediscover his passions, re-engage with family and friends, and maintain an exercise regimen. And with hope on the horizon, both his pain and function have improved.

The pain field grew not only in America but also around the world, and the quest for pain management as a fundamental human right was global. One must ask, then, why the United States was the only country in which the change in attitude led to a prescription opioid epidemic, and why the United States continues to consume most of the world's prescription opioids. What was it that protected other countries? Probably the most straightforward contributing factor is the difference in the way healthcare is provided. The United States is the only wealthy country that does not have universal healthcare. Because other wealthy countries do have universal healthcare, they have gatekeepers. For example, primary care physicians hold all the medical records for their allocated patients and manage their medications and access to specialty care. Decisions about what treatments are offered tend to be made at the national level, not locally or by private insurers. This means patients in these countries generally have less control of or ability to demand treatments, and less sense of entitlement. Pharmaceutical representatives have less access to prescribers. At the same time, nationally derived treatment decisions are more likely to be strongly evidence-based. Because it has relatively strong evidence supporting it, multidisciplinary pain care may be more readily available. Because chronic opioid therapy does not have a strong evidence base, it is less likely to be utilized. Poorer countries, with less well-organized healthcare systems, tend to have strict opioid controls, which provides protection from misuse but is also the reason that poorer countries often lack even palliative care.

Much more complex than healthcare system issues are the cultural issues that go a long way toward explaining why America has been so badly affected. America is a young country founded on the ideals of rebels who rejected the mores of the countries they came from. America always tries to do better, believes in its ability to improve, and rejects the status quo.

Behind it all lies perhaps the most famous sentence in history: "We hold these truths to be self-evident, that all men are created equal, that they are endowed by their creator with certain inalienable Rights, that among these are Life, Liberty and pursuit of Happiness." In the countries the framers of the Declaration of Independence had left behind, few people imagined they had a right to personal happiness. More likely they were grateful to God and country, and their duty was to them, not to self. In the words of historian Richard Davenport Hines, "Only in the USA was personal happiness, or individual fulfillment, enshrined with such formality as a human entitlement; only there were national beliefs, values and norms centered on this idea of inalienable emotional rights."[33(p125)]

Before ideas about a right to pain relief were proposed, John Bonica advanced the idea that it was not necessary to suffer chronic pain, that medicine could intervene to reduce it. America led the world in developing pain clinics, and Americans fully embraced the idea that it was not necessary to suffer prolonged pain. By the time a right to pain relief was proposed, the argument for pain relief had begun to include the idea that not only was pain relief desirable, but failure to provide it was harmful. In the words of Michael Cousins:

> There is ample documentation now that persistent pain, even in the subacute phase after surgery, and in association with childbirth, can cause severe psychological and even psychiatric effects, which might be persistent. There is also some extraordinary emerging evidence that persisting pain causes persisting physical effects involving pathophysiology of the nervous system itself.[25(p541)]

What is missing from this description is that neuroadaptations to pain are not necessarily bad, and in fact pain exists so that the person can adapt to the environment and survive.[34] But imagine the mindset of Americans, pioneers by nature, when they become convinced that severe pain should not be tolerated.

Another way in which the American character increased its vulnerability to overuse of opioids for the treatment of pain relates to attitudes to drug use. It is paradoxical that America became the greatest proponent of opioid pain treatment, while it has also been among the greatest opponents of drug use outside medicine. American drug regulations have been especially draconian. The full force of its Drug Enforcement Agency (DEA) is felt throughout the world. More Americans are in jail for drug offenses (even minor drug offenses) than in any other country. There is much support for abstinence treatment of drug abuse despite high rates of recidivism. Jail is used as a substitute for addiction treatment. And despite efforts to frame addiction as a disease (something not under the person's control), drug use and addiction are still widely disparaged.

The resulting "opiophobia" has been used by pain advocates to argue for the removal of restrictions on prescribing and for the universal monitoring of pain. "Intractable pain" statutes began to be written, asserting the right of patients to receive opioids without limits, and the protection of clinicians prescribing for pain.[35] In 2001, the Joint Commission for the Accreditation of Healthcare Organizations (JCAHO) introduced pain standards into quality metrics mandating that pain be assessed and treated.[36] The need for such aggressive measures to impose pain management as a requirement was rarely needed in other countries, largely because opioid use was not disparaged to the same extent.

Finally, America is much more prone to the influence of the pharmaceutical industry than other countries, not least because America is a wealthy country with a huge population and vast buying power. Most companies with opioid products are highly active in the United States because of the size of the market, none more so than Purdue Pharma. Purdue Pharma's marketing tactics have been quite brilliant, and very effective. Unfortunately for Purdue, their tactics have also bordered on illegal, and the company was forced to declare bankruptcy in 2019 under the burden of legal cases against it (said to be over 2000). But not before their successful marketing resulted in massive sales for their drug OxyContin, with their educational message seeping into the medical community's understanding of opioid treatment in general. Purdue had a large educational department, sponsored postgraduate medical education widely, underwrote patient advocacy groups and pain societies, and supported the teaching activities and research of clinicians and scientists who were "on message." As is now well known, Purdue exaggerated the benefits and trivialized the risks of its products, leading to blind overuse and to the U.S. opioid epidemic.

There is, of course, no way of disengaging America's opioid epidemic from its so-called deaths of despair, those deaths arising through suicide and the health consequences of drug and alcohol use. The opioid epidemic is reflected in the deaths of despair and reflected by them. Overdose deaths contribute to

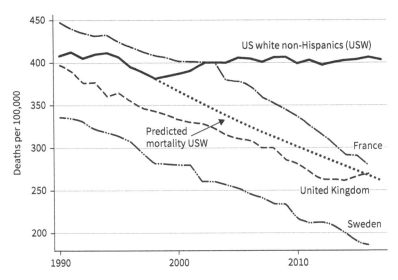

Figure 3.4. Age-adjusted mortality rates, ages 45–54, for US white non-Hispanics (USW), France, UK and Sweden, and a predicted mortality for USW. A counterfactual that assumes the mortality rate for USW would continue falling at 2% per year after 1998. Authors' calculations using CDC data and Human Mortality Database. From: Deaths of Despair and the Future of Capitalism. Anne Case and Angus Deaton. Princeton University Press 2020, with permission.

deaths of despair, and despair contributes to pain and its treatment with opioids. As a result, international life expectancy rankings for Americans have fallen behind other wealthy countries over the past decade.[37-39] For the first time since mortality rates have been recorded, mortality rates for white non-Hispanic males are increasing instead of declining, a phenomenon that is not occurring in any other country (Figures 3.4 and 3.5). The rise in deaths in America is affecting particularly less-educated White Americans.

These deaths have been attributed to drug overdoses, suicides, and drug- and alcohol-related disease.[39] Case and Deaton, quoting Emile Durkheim's *Le suicide: Etude de sociologie* (1897), have proposed that despair arises in societies that can no longer provide their members an environment in which they can live a meaningful life. They attribute the despair to loss of meaning more than to poverty or job loss per se:

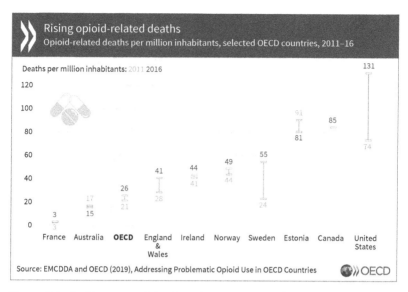

Figure 3.5. Problem prescribing from the Organisation for Economic Co-operation and Development (OECD) paper, "Addressing Problematic Opioid Use in OECD Countries," page 2: Presentations and Key Data.

European Monitoring Center for Drugs and Drugs Addiction and OECD, 2019: https://www.oecd.org/health/addressing-problematic-opioid-use-in-oecd-countries-a18286f0-en.htm

In spite of the austerity in some countries, or lack of it in others, there was (and is) no epidemic of deaths of despair in Europe; the slowdowns and reversals in mortality rates in the United States have no general counterpart in Europe. Indeed, between 2007 and 2013, while unemployment rates in Greece and Spain more than tripled—to the point where more than a quarter of the population was unemployed—life expectancy was rising more rapidly than in most other European countries.

Americans had such hope that they would lead better and better lives, generation after generation. The post-WWII years sustained that hope. After the war, a few generations of Americans did improve their standards of living, and the expectation that their children would do better than they did was borne out. Maybe the idea that their gains would continue forever was a naïve hope, carried on the crest of enthusiasm of a new nation promising individual happiness. But what happened was that the wealth went to the few, and many of those who had lived comfortable lives working for companies that became vulnerable were cast aside when those enterprises were no longer needed. There was less of a social safety net than exists in most other wealthy countries, partly because Americans endorse individualism and non-reliance on governments, even if they need help. The young moved away from decimated small communities to seek a better life in urban communities, and activities such as participation in family dinners, entertaining friends at home, going to church, and belonging to clubs and unions began to slip away for lack of energy and reward. In their book *Deaths of Despair and the Future of Capitalism*, Case and Deaton attribute American deaths of despair to five factors:

1. The American healthcare system, which they submit is causing the deaths of despair by draining the economy
2. The erosion of community
3. America's history of race relations and the shadow of slavery
4. Lack of social protection
5. The dependence of American politics on large sums of campaign finance and lobbying.

One thing that has been learned since the early Bonica years is that chronic pain is not a simple reflection of damage to the painful body part, something that can be easily fixed. Even though it may be experienced as physical in nature (bodily pain), it has deep ties to emotional distress. This makes people with chronic pain susceptible to drug use, abuse, suicide, and overdose deaths. Chronic pain may be no more prevalent in the United States than in other countries, but the context in which it arises, through broken lives and loss of hope, and the health system in which it is cared for, full of pharmaceutical and procedural entrepreneurs, made Americans especially susceptible to high opioid use and bad opioid outcomes.

Conclusion

In this chapter, we have described how a right to pain relief was established. This occurred largely in the 20th century in parallel with an explosion in the growth and diversity of medical tools available to treat pain. Establishing a right to pain relief at the end of life was a first step toward declaring that all humans are entitled to relief of their pain. Some palliative care experts even called for a right to relief through opioid treatment. Professional advocates for liberalized opioid treatment of chronic pain generally fell short of explicitly declaring a right to pain relief through opioid treatment, although pharmaceutical marketing materials implied that this right had been established. This right to relief of chronic pain was understood as reduction in a pain intensity score. This relief was to be accomplished through titration of opioid doses to this effect.

This right to pain relief was part of the grand effort to control our fate in this world through medical interventions. Medicine replaced religion as our primary explanation for pain. It delivered on its promise of controlling pain thought previously to be necessary and inevitable. Through control of pain during surgery and pain at the end of life, medicine pushed back the boundary between escapable and inescapable pain. It hoped to do the same with chronic pain. To understand why this effort failed, we must look further into how chronic pain has been conceived as a public health and clinical problem.

References

1. Papper EM. *Romance, Poetry, and Surgical Sleep: Literature Influences Medicine.* Greenwood Press; 1995.
2. Sykes WS. *Essays on the First Hundred Years of Anaesthesia.* Wood Library, Museum of Anesthesiology; 1960.
3. Mott V. Successful ligature of the common iliac artery. *Am J Med Sci.* 1827;1:156–161.
4. Weir Mitchell S. *Injuries of the Nerves and Their Consequences.* J. B. Lippincott; 1872.
5. Melzack R, Wall PD. Pain mechanisms: a new theory. *Science.* 1965;150:971–979.
6. Merskey H. *An Investigation of Pain in Psychological Illness.* Oxford, DM thesis; 1964.
7. United Nations. Universal Declaration of Human Rights. 1948. https://www.un.org/en/about-us/universal-declaration-of-human-rights
8. Ogden J, Ambrose L, Khadra A, et al. A questionnaire study of GPs' and patients' beliefs about the different components of patient centredness. *Patient Educ Couns.* 2002;47:223–227.

9. Foley KM. Testimony before Congress on medical issues related to physician-assisted suicide. 1996.

10. Bonica JJ, Ventafridda V. *Advances in Pain Research and Therapy, Vol. 2: International Symposium on Pain of Advanced Cancer.* Raven Press; 1979.

11. Gwyther L, Brennan F, Harding R. Advancing palliative care as a human right. *J Pain Symptom Manage.* 2009;38:767–774.

12. Burt RA. The Supreme Court speaks—not assisted suicide but a constitutional right to palliative care. *N Engl J Med.* 1997;337:1234–1236.

13. Gostin LO. Deciding life and death in the courtroom. From Quinlan to Cruzan, Glucksberg, and Vacco—a brief history and analysis of constitutional protection of the "right to die." *JAMA.* 1997;278:1523–1528.

14. Mpanga Sebuyira L, Mwangi-Powell F, Pereira J, Spence C. The Cape Town Palliative Care Declaration: home-grown solutions for sub-Saharan Africa. *J Palliat Med.* 2003;6:341–343.

15. National Hospice and Palliative Care Associations. The Korea Declaration. Report of the second global summit of National Hospice and Palliative Care Associations, Seoul, Korea, 2005. http://www/eplc-observatory.net/global/pdf/NHPCA_2.pdf

16. European Association for Palliatve Care. The Budapest Commitments. http://www.eapcnet.org/congresses/Budapest2007/Budapest2007Commitments.htm

17. International Association for Hospice and Pallaitve Care and the Worldwide Pallative Care Alliance. Joint declaration and statement of commitment on palliative care and pain treatment as human rights. http://www.hospicecare.com/resources/pain_pallcare_hr/docs/jdsc.pdf

18. Special Rapporteurs on the question of torture and the right of everyone to the highest attainable standard of physical and mental health. Letter to Mr D Best, vice-chairperson of the commission on narcotic drugs, December 10, 2008. http://www.ihra.net/Assets/1384/1/SpecialRapporteursLettertoCND012009.pdf

19. American Academy of Pain Medicine and the American Pain Society. The use of opioids for the treatment of chronic pain. *Clin J Pain.* 1997;13:6–8.

20. Joranson DE, Gilson AM, Dahl JL, Haddox JD. Pain medicine, controlled substances, and state medical board policy: a decade of change. *J Pain Symptom Manage.* 2002;23:138–147.

21. Peter Ward Fey "The Opium War" (1840–42) (1975).

22. Bruce CA. *Report on the Manufacture of Tea and on the Extent and Produce of the Tea Plantations in Assam.* Calcutta; 1839.

23. Portenoy RK, Foley KM. Chronic use of opioid analgesics in non-malignant pain: report of 38 cases. *Pain*. 1986;25: 171–86.

24. Melzack R. The tragedy of needless pain. *Sci Am*. 1990;262:27–33.

25. Cousins MJ. Pain: the past, present, and future of anesthesiology? The E. A. Rovenstine Memorial Lecture. *Anesthesiology*. 1999;91:538–551.

26. Cousins MJ. Relief of acute pain: a basic human right? *Med J Aust*. 2000;172:3–4.

27. Cousins MJ, Brennan F, Carr DB. Pain relief: a universal human right. *Pain*. 2004;112:1–4.

28. Brennan F, Carr DB, Cousins M. Pain management: a fundamental human right. *Anesth Analg*. 2007;105:205–221.

29. White PF, Kehlet H. Improving pain management: are we jumping from the frying pan into the fire? *Anesth Analg*. 2007;105:10–12.

30. Paulozzi LJ, Budnitz DS, Xi Y. Increasing deaths from opioid analgesics in the United States. *Pharmacoepidemiol Drug Saf*. 2006;15:618–627.

31. DeWeerdt S. The natural history of an epidemic. *Nature*. 2019;573:S10–S12.

32. Quinones S. *Dreamland: The True Tale of America's Opiate Epidemic*. Bloomsbury Press; 2016.

33. Davenport-Hines T. *The Pursuit of Oblivion: A Global History of Narcotics*. Weidenfeld and Nicolson; 2001.

34. Loeser JD. The tragedy of painless needs. *Pain Res Manag*. 2000;5:228–232.

35. Joranson DE, Gilson AM. State intractable pain policy: Current status. *APS Bull*. 1997;7:7–9.

36. Joint Commission on Accreditation of Healthcare Organizations. Pain management standards. 2001. https://www.jointcommission.org/-/media/tjc/docume nts/resources/pain-management/2001_pain_standardspdf.pdf

37. Ho JY. The contemporary American drug overdose epidemic in international perspective. *Pop Devel Rev*. 2019;45:7–40.

38. Ho JY, Hendi AS. Recent trends in life expectancy across high income countries: retrospective observational study. *BMJ*. 2018;362:k2562.

39. Case A, Deaton A. Rising morbidity and mortality in midlife among white non-Hispanic Americans in the 21st century. *Proc Natl Acad Sci USA*. 2015;112:15078–15083.

4
Chronic pain as a disease

Without pain, the world would be an impossibly dangerous place.
Institute of Medicine report, *Relieving Pain in America*

Introduction: how big a problem is chronic pain?

Opioid prescribing has been justified as an answer to the problem of chronic pain. Chronic pain can be understood as a clinical problem of individual patients or as a public health problem of a population of patients. But these understandings of individuals and populations with chronic pain are not independent. Epidemiology helps define the nature as well as the extent of the clinical problem of chronic pain. The U.S. National Institutes of Health (NIH) defines epidemiology as follows:

> Epidemiology is the branch of medical science that investigates all the factors that determine the presence or absence of diseases and disorders. Epidemiological research helps us to understand how many people have a disease or disorder, if those numbers are changing, and how the disorder affects our society and our economy.[1]

Epidemiology originated in the study of epidemics. In this chapter, we will examine how epidemiology has shaped our understanding of chronic pain as a public health problem and as a clinical problem. The epidemiology of chronic pain has focused on linking chronic pain to other chronic diseases. This certainly makes sense when chronic pain is considered a symptom of other diseases like osteoarthritis or multiple sclerosis. Chronic pain is also linked with other diseases as risk factors such as obesity. But medical professionals have gone beyond this. In general, professionals have used the template of chronic disease to understand chronic pain. This template highlights biomedical causes and remedies for chronic pain while throwing social causes of and remedies for chronic pain into the shadows. It has been a crucial part of the medicalization of chronic pain.

Some experts have argued that the opioid epidemic can only be addressed by simultaneously addressing the "pain epidemic" where "millions of Americans were suffering needlessly from untreated pain."[2,3] In her 2014 book *A Nation in Pain,* science journalist Judy Foreman argued that "lack of adequate pain control is one of the most urgent health problems in America.... America is in the midst of a chronic pain epidemic."[4] In its 2011 report on *Relieving Pain in America,* the Institute of Medicine (IOM) cited the following reasons for the rising rates of chronic pain: aging of the population, rising prevalence of obesity, increased survival after serious injury or illness, and increasing outpatient surgery. They also suggest that "greater public understanding of chronic pain syndromes and the development of new treatments may cause many people who have not sought help or who previously gave up on treatment to reenter the health care system."[5] A number of specific studies of low back pain are cited in the IOM report, including a study from North Carolina that showed an increase from 1992 to 2006 in chronic low back pain from 4% to 10% of the total population, with greater increases in women and middle-aged men.[6] A national study from the Veterans Affairs health system is cited, showing an annualized increase in the prevalence of low back pain of about 5% per year.[7] National data from the National Health and Nutrition Examination Survey (NHANES) survey are also cited, showing that the percentage of men reporting pain in the previous month increased from 19% in 1999–2000 to 25% in 2003–2004 and the percent of women reporting pain in the previous month increased from 25% in 1999–2000 to 30% in 2003–2004.[8]

These are significant increases in the reporting of back pain and pain in any given month, though these figures do not come close to the quadrupling of opioid prescriptions seen in the United States during this time. Some other high-income countries have seen increases in opioid prescribing (Australia, Canada, Denmark, Finland, Germany, Sweden, and the United Kingdom), but these have generally been smaller and slower increases than in the United States and have involved less potent opioids. Ho has recently summarized the comparisons with other high-income countries that have aging populations: "Drug overdose mortality is now 3.5 times higher on average in the US than other high-income countries. It is over 27 times higher than in Italy and Japan, which have the lowest drug overdose death rates, and 60 percent higher than in Finland and Sweden, the comparator countries with the next highest death rates." These data suggest that, even if the prevalence of chronic pain is increasing, this increase is not nearly enough to explain or justify the increase in American opioid prescribing.

We will argue that changes in our concepts and values about pain and opioids were much more important than increases in the prevalence of chronic pain in creating the opioid epidemic. Why did we decide in the 1990s that "millions of Americans were suffering needlessly from untreated pain"? We reviewed part of the explanation in our last chapter: With the help of pharmaceutical companies and doctors, Americans came to see opioids as safer and more effective for chronic pain than before. Advocates argued that our willingness to treat pain had been constrained by irrational fears of opioid pain treatment or "opiophobia." In this chapter, we will examine how Americans came to see any prevalent pain as "undertreated pain." We will need to examine concepts used in the evolving science of pain epidemiology to understand what it means for pain to be undertreated because it is not clear what a normal or tolerable level of pain should be. Zero pain is not a viable goal (see the chapter epigraph). Because some pain is necessary for life and because all pain treatments come with a cost to health and well-being, we face significant conceptual and value challenges in characterizing and quantifying the medical problem of pain. Our thesis in this chapter is that to understand the epidemic of opioids dispensed as pain treatment, we must first understand how ambiguities about the status of pain as a medical problem have been addressed.

Ted Kasin, part 1

Ted Kasin is a 48-year-old married White male who presents with a 6-month history of severe recurrent back pain. He had a previous episode of back pain 4 years ago after a workplace injury at the auto assembly plant where he works on the line attaching fenders. This resolved after 6 weeks off work, physical therapy, and non-opioid medications. His current episode of back pain started a month after he was laid off from the auto plant. A day after raking his yard, he woke up with severe back pain. He says that this pain is more intense than his previous back pain (this pain is 9/10, the previous pain was 7/10) and has not responded to the ibuprofen he used last time. He asks for some Vicodin (hydrocodone).

Epidemiological surveys of pain: quantifying pain as a public health problem

If pain is to be approached and addressed as a medical problem, it must be identified and tracked in the population as a public health issue. In its 2011 report *Relieving Pain In America*, the IOM famously stated that 100 million U.S. adults had chronic pain conditions at an annual cost of $560 to $635 billion.[5] On what basis does this report say that 100 million adults have chronic pain? How were these cost estimates derived? What do these imply about clinical treatments and public health measures for this problem of chronic pain?

When we were in medical school in the 1970s and 1980s, we were taught that pain is a symptom of disease or injury. Our main clinical task and our primary responsibility toward patients with pain was to accurately diagnose and treat that disease or injury that was causing their pain. That treatment would serve to reduce the risks to life and limb posed by the disease and provide the most potent and enduring relief of pain to the patient. We still remember being taught not to allow the patient's demands for pain relief to distract us from this primary task of diagnosing and treating disease. This was especially true in the case of acute abdominal pain, where the character, location, and response of the pain to various physical exam maneuvers was considered crucial to the accurate diagnosis of its cause, and these signs could be masked by pain treatment. It was important, for example, to determine if the cause was appendicitis, for which surgery may be needed, or gastroenteritis, for which watchful waiting is fine. In addition to focusing clinical attention, the understanding of pain as a symptom of disease gave pain a clear, if limited, place in medical theory and practice: *Pain is a medical problem because its cause is disease.* Defining disease can be complex and contentious. Here we will operate with a standard definition of disease, such as the following from the *Merriam-Webster Dictionary*: "a condition of the living animal or plant body or of one of its parts that impairs normal functioning and is typically manifested by distinguishing signs and symptoms."[9] We only add that in modern medicine, disease is an objective condition that precedes and causes a patient's subjective symptoms.

John Bonica railed against the idea that pain is merely a symptom of disease.[10] He argued that this symptom idea did not capture the experience or the significance of the pain for the patient. And for Bonica, this shortfall was especially true for chronic pain, defined as pain that extends beyond the healing time of any associated disease or injury. With chronic pain, there is often no causal disease to diagnose and treat. This type of pain is thus both a medical and evolutionary anomaly. It often does not point to disease that can be treated. Even more puzzling, it does not appear to serve any tissue protective function. What tissues are chronic headaches or chronic low back pain protecting? What evolutionary purpose is served by pain that is not needed to protect the painful body part?

Pain, especially chronic pain without clear association to disease or injury, remains marginal in medical science. Despite pain being one of the most common reasons that patients consult physicians, there is still no NIH institute devoted to the study of pain. The tools that medicine uses to treat pain beyond the treatment of disease are growing, but still limited. It is not surprising that when medicine was called upon to seriously assess and treat chronic pain by the palliative care community in the 1990s, it turned to one of its oldest, most potent, and most reliable analgesics: opioids.

As mentioned, the IOM's 2011 report called for "a cultural transformation in the way clinicians and the public view pain and its treatment."[5] This transformation includes multiple facets, but its most important meaning in the report is clear: "Understanding chronic pain as a disease means that it requires direct treatment, rather than being sidelined while clinicians attempt to identify some underlying condition that may have caused it."[5] We are thus urged to move from understanding pain as a symptom of disease to pain as a disease unto itself. But are these our only two options for framing pain as a problem? Chronic pain could be considered a condition, like frailty, that is neither a symptom nor a disease. It could also be considered a universal part of the human experience, like suffering.

The clinical significance of calling chronic pain a disease is also unclear, for what does it mean to treat pain as a disease during a clinic visit? Does this mean more or less diagnostic imaging, more or less medication prescription? It is also unclear what it means to treat pain as a disease from a public health perspective. In the 2011 IOM report, the public health burden of chronic pain in the United States is quantified in terms of its associated costs and its population prevalence. There is also mention of the "moral imperative for effective pain management." But what is not addressed is the question of threshold: When does chronic pain become a public health problem? When does chronic pain need medical treatment? The IOM report mentions "inadequate pain prevention, assessment and treatment" but also "unrealistic patient expectations" about pain treatment. We are not told how to reconcile these contradictory admonitions.

It is not true that all pain is a medical problem. Pain is essential to human life. As the IOM report itself stated, "Without pain, the world would be an impossibly dangerous place." It is necessary to set a threshold at which pain becomes a medical problem. For a more traditional disease like diabetes, this medical threshold is set at the point at which impaired glucose metabolism causes mortality or at the point where impaired glucose metabolism produces serious organ morbidity like renal failure and blindness. But pain does not have these clear associations with mortality and morbidity. Another type of threshold is necessary.

Michael Von Korff, one of the foremost chronic pain epidemiologists, has questioned the 100 million number from the IOM report. He explains that this figure was derived from the World Mental Health Survey in response to a question about the presence of any chronic pain in the past 12 months.[11] This question "was to compare the prevalence of common chronic pain conditions in different countries, not to estimate the percentage of the population who might need treatment for chronic pain." The World Mental Health Survey did not, for example, differentiate moderate or severe chronic pain from mild chronic pain. Von Korff asks, "Is there a moral imperative for health care professionals to treat all persons with chronic pain irrespective of its severity or of the potential benefits from therapeutic interventions?"[11] "I think not" is his answer, and we agree. He adds a crucial explanation: "Human suffering alone does not confer a moral imperative for medical intervention."[11] He adds, "A moral imperative for treatment is based on the potential for treatment benefits to exceed harms and costs."[11] We also agree with this statement and will return to it later in this chapter. But first we will consider the various thresholds that have been proposed for determining when pain becomes a medical problem and warrants medical treatment.

How do we measure the need for medical treatment of chronic pain?

Quantitative pain severity as an index of medical need and treatment success

We intuitively understand pain as an experience. If we are pressed to describe what kind of experience pain is, we tend to describe it as a sensory experience with a specific intensity. As pain neuroscientist Don Price stated, "If pain is defined as an experience, then the scientific study of pain ultimately has to study and even measure that experience."[12] The measurement of the pain sensation is generally how pain assessment has been mandated and implemented in clinical practice. It is consistent with our post-Cartesian modern mechanical understanding of how pain experiences are produced within our body. The pain sensation concept is favored by patients and advocates who closely link pain and injury, conceptualizing chronic pain as a peripherally produced aversive sensation imposed on an innocent person. Although this understanding may not be scientifically valid, clinically useful, or productively implemented in policy, it has been at the core of our modern concept of pain, so we must try to understand its strengths and limitations.

In his 1995 Presidential Address to the American Pain Society (APS), neurosurgeon James Campbell famously called for American medicine to adopt pain as the "fifth vital sign" alongside the four traditional vital signs of pulse, blood pressure, temperature, and respiration rate.[13] After claiming that the mission of the APS is to strive for quality of life, "something that is more precious than simple perpetuation of life," he argued that "[n]eedless suffering from pain is not acceptable."[13] He quoted James Mill, the Scottish utilitarian philosopher: "The lot of every human being is determined by his pains and pleasures, and … his happiness corresponds with the degree in which his pleasures are great and his pains are small."[13] Campbell argued that pain control is essential, not just for good postoperative care, but also for "acute exacerbations of back pain, with rheumatoid arthritis, and with myriad other diseases."[13] This reminds us that the medical approach to the problem of pain is aligned with the utilitarian approach discussed in Chapter 1 and properly understood as a subset of that approach.

Rather than putting "the patient in a position of seeming to ask for a favor of the primary care doctor to get adequate pain control for a simple backache,"[13] Campbell argued we should routinely assess and treat pain: "Patient-controlled analgesia teaches us that an incredibly simple 0-to-10 scale can be used easily to measure suffering from pain. We tell the patient to imagine that 10 is the worst pain you can imagine having and that 0 is no pain at all." After drawing an analogy with the routine assessment of vital signs, he argued:

> We should consider pain the *fifth vital sign*. When a patient says, "My pain is a 9," this is like running a fever or like having a hypotensive crisis or atrial fibrillation. We know how to treat most pain.... We know how to take pain at a level of 9 and lower it to 3.... If pain were assessed with the same zeal as other vital signs are, it would have a much better chance of being treated properly. We need to train doctors and nurses to treat pain as a vital sign. *Quality care* means that pain is measured. *Quality of care* means that pain is treated.[13]

Campbell made clear that this vital sign concept is not only for postoperative pain: "Chronic pain can be measured on a 0-to-10 scale as easily as acute pain. If pain is scaled high, this is a vital sign that the patient requires treatment, regardless of whether the patient has postoperative pain or more enduring chronic pain." He went on to state that misinformation about addiction and fears of regulatory action have made us blind to the fact that "a patient did not necessarily have to have cancer to derive long-term alleviation of pain from use of opioids." He concluded with the suggestion that "these guidelines be used as part of the overall guidelines for hospital accreditation."

In 1998, the Veterans Affairs Administration enacted a national strategy to improve pain management. This strategy required providers to assess a patient's pain intensity, as measured on a 0-to-10 numeric rating scale (NRS) (Figure 4.1), and record this in their electronic medical record. It was also noted that "a pain score of 4 or higher would trigger a comprehensive pain assessment and prompt intervention." In 2001, the body responsible for accrediting U.S. healthcare organizations (now the Joint Commission, previously known as Joint Commission on the Accreditation of Health Care Organizations [JCAHO]) followed the suggestion of a group of pain advocates and mandated national pain assessment and management standards.[14]

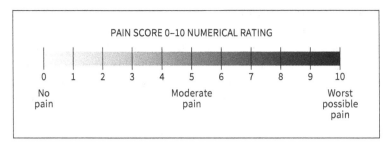

Figure 4.1. 0-to-10 numerical rating scale for pain

While JCAHO did not specifically require use of the 0-to-10 NRS, this became the most common way that the mandate was implemented.

This pain *assessment* strategy was transformed into a pain *treatment* strategy through combination with the "titrate to effect" principle. This principle had been formulated in acute pain, cancer pain, and end-of-life care. It taught that, unlike with most other prescribed medications, there is no pre-specified correct dose of opioids that is right for all patients. The correct dose of opioid is whatever dose provides pain relief, as measured by a pain intensity scale. This principle had been disseminated as part of the World Health Organization (WHO) stepladder approach to the management of cancer pain.[15] Step 1 includes non-opioid analgesics. Step 2 includes Step 1 plus weak opioid analgesics. Step 3 includes Step 2 plus strong opioid analgesics. Each step also includes adjuvant therapies. The underlying principle of the stepladder approach is that analgesic doses and strengths should be escalated as necessary to reduce the pain level as much as possible.

But does pain intensity measurement provide a good assessment of an individual's burden of chronic pain? The experience of chronic pain is not simply the perception of an aversive sensation of some specific intensity; it is a disruption in one's ability to live the life one desires. How necessary is a reduction in pain intensity for a reduction in suffering? Classically, pain is understood as an experience that arises in the body, while suffering arises within the person. In modern medicine, pain and suffering are often conflated: Severe physical pain is equated with extreme suffering. Yet intense postoperative pain can be tolerable because we know it will end, and the intense pain of childbirth may be tempered by joy. But pain that has no meaning or known end may produce great suffering, not only because of its intensity, but also because it poses a threat to one's integrity.[16]

We assume that more intense pain is less tolerable. Recent research suggests this is generally true, but subject to considerable variation. Markman and colleagues assessed 663 primary care patients with an analgesic prescription or a chronic pain visit diagnosis. They were asked to complete a standard 0-to-10 NRS of pain intensity and to answer another question: "Is your pain tolerable?" In the mild range of pain intensity (1–3/10), no patients rated their pain as intolerable. In the moderate range (4–6/10), 19% of patients rated their pain as intolerable. In the severe range (7–10/10), 53%, slightly more than half, rated their pain as intolerable.[17] These results suggest that tolerability is related to intensity, but is distinct from it. Tolerability is a more direct reflection of a patient's need for treatment, but a less direct assessment of their pain sensation. Tolerability is a more personal form of pain assessment than intensity.

Tolerability is not the only clinically important feature of pain that shows a variable relationship with pain intensity. Adams and colleagues studied 189 patients with high pain intensity (7–10/10) who were prescribed long-term opioid therapy for chronic musculoskeletal pain from two healthcare systems. Within this group, 16% had low pain interference with daily tasks, 39% had moderate interference, and 44% had high interference. The group that had low pain interference (despite high pain intensity) had less depression and anxiety, less pain catastrophizing, a better quality of life, and greater self-efficacy (confidence) for managing pain.[18] These results suggest that the effect that pain has on patients' lives is determined by factors beyond pain intensity. These factors that determine the tolerability of pain are features of the patient in pain rather than features of the pain sensation.

Pain intensity measures are not only a poor indicator of the need for chronic pain treatment but are also a poor indicator of whether pain treatment is succeeding. Many of our most evidence-based, U.S. Food and Drug Administration (FDA)-approved medications for chronic pain (e.g., duloxetine, pregabalin) don't reduce pain intensity more than 1 point on the 0-to-10 scale in controlled clinical trials. Impressive reductions in the intensity of chronic pain can be produced with opioid therapy in the short term. But in a year-long randomized trial, opioids reduced chronic back or joint pain no more than non-opioid analgesics.[19] Further evidence that reported pain intensity is a poor indicator of the success of pain treatment comes from studies of patients with free access to opioid medications for labor pain or cancer pain who chose not to lower their pain intensity to "acceptable" levels due to a desire to remain alert and communicative.[20,21] These patients clearly considered factors beyond pain intensity in determining what constitutes adequate or successful treatment. In fact, three-fourths of patients who are prescribed sustained-release opioids for chronic pain never refill the prescription.[22] This is presumably because the side effects are not worth the pain reduction achieved.

Furthermore, it is not clear whether FDA-approved chronic pain treatments produce their benefit primarily by decreasing pain intensity. Although many patients understand chronic pain to be the cause of their many problems in living, clinical treatments for chronic pain often improve sleep, mood, or functional status *before* they improve pain. We have demonstrated this in a large sample of patients attending the University of Washington Center for Pain Relief.[23] A variety of research studies suggest that chronic pain treatments affect reported pain intensity indirectly or secondarily. The effect of pregabalin on the eight subscales of the Short Form Health Survey (SF-36) general health status measure is only partially mediated by pain reduction.[24] Other analyses demonstrate that pregabalin pain relief is preceded and predicted by sleep improvement.[25] In another study, improvements in both pain and depression after 2 weeks of venlafaxine treatment predicted the amount of improvement in pain at 6 weeks.[26] Multidisciplinary pain rehabilitation programs and cognitive–behavioral treatments (CBT) of chronic pain often produce earlier and more marked reductions in pain-related disability than pain intensity.[27,28] The 2020 Cochrane review of CBT trials reports that CBT reduces pain and distress and disability by only small or very small amounts.[29] Thus, many of our best chronic pain treatments do not affect pain intensity ratings substantially or primarily. This suggests that pain intensity reduction may not be the primary or sole goal for chronic pain treatment.

Disability as an index of the burden of chronic pain

More recent studies of chronic pain prevalence in the United States and around the world have focused on the disability associated with chronic pain as the best measure of the burden of chronic pain for individuals and popu-lations. Population estimates of the prevalence of chronic pain in the United States have ranged from 11% to 40%, with considerable variation among population subgroups.[30] The lack of reliable prevalence estimates makes it difficult to characterize the public health problem posed by chronic pain or to aim prevention and treatment efforts appropriately. Therefore, the 2016 National Pain Strategy called for more precise estimates of the prevalence of chronic pain and the prevalence of serious chronic pain that warrants med-ical treatment.

Ted Kasin, part 2

Ted Kasin describes his current pain intensity as a 9 on a 10-point scale. He is asked to describe how that has limited his activity. He explains that he was offered back his old job at the auto plant a month ago, but he was unable to return to work due to his back pain. Furthermore, since the back pain began while he was laid off, he is not eligible for time loss through workers' compensation. He also describes decreased ability to do house-hold chores, to participate in hobbies like motorcycle riding, and even to watch movies with his wife, Connie.

Based on analyses of the 2016 National Interview Survey Data, the Centers for Disease Control and Prevention (CDC) has estimated that 20% of U.S. adults (50 million) have chronic pain and 8% have "high-impact" chronic pain (20 million) that limits their life and work activi-ties.[31] Chronic pain was defined as pain on most days in the past 6 months. High-impact chronic pain was defined as chronic pain that limited life or work activities on most days during the past 6 months. Both chronic pain and high-impact chronic pain are more common among women, adults no longer working, adults in poverty, and rural residents. Adults with at least a bachelor's degree had less chronic pain and high-impact chronic pain. Although non-Hispanic White adults had more chronic pain that other ethnic groups, they did not have more high-impact chronic pain. In a separate study of patients receiving care at Kaiser Permanente in Oregon and Washington, only 2.4% of patients with mild chronic pain and 2.7% of patients with bothersome chronic pain were receiving long-term opioid therapy, but 17.7% of patients with high-impact chronic pain were receiving long-term opioids.[32]

The current diagnosis of high-impact chronic pain is based on "most days" or "every day" responses to the question: "Over the past 3 months, how often did pain limit your life or work activities?" This focus on pain-related activity interference and functional impairment as an index of pain burden is an advance on pain intensity because it situates pain as a problem within life, rather than treating it as a separate sensation. It is an improved measure of medical treatment need for patients with chronic pain because it subordinates pain reduction to health and functional improvement. Patients with high-impact chronic pain have reported higher rates of "limits doing household chores," "limits using transportation," limits leisure activities," and "limits getting out with friends or family" than patients with mild or bothersome chronic pain.[32]

If the focus on the intensity of the pain sensation can be called an "internalist" account of the experience and burden of chronic pain, the focus on pain-associated disability can be called an "externalist" account. Internalist accounts, like that of Descartes, assume that all the phenomena relevant to understanding the experience of pain occur within the boundaries of the body. These include tissue damage, sensations, and the physiological processes that connect these. Externalist accounts, on the other hand, consider phenomena outside the body as relevant to the experience and burden of pain. Disability concerns the capacity of the body to interact productively with the outside environment. It is obviously determined by features of that external environment, such as the nature of available work, what activities are necessary for daily life, and what work support is provided for people who are injured. The internalist approach is focused in a classically biomedical manner, with attention limited to processes inside the body that are readily available to clinical examination. The externalist approach directs the clinician's attention outside the exam room to the circumstances of the patient's life. It suggests a broader array of social interventions to address the burden of chronic pain for individuals and populations.

Using disability to quantify the burden of chronic pain across countries

Defining the burden of non-fatal chronic conditions has been one of the main goals of the Global Burden of Disease (GBD) study launched by WHO in the 1990s.[33] The 2010 GBD study sought to quantify the years lived with disability (YLDs) for persons with 289 different diseases and injuries.[34] The leading causes of YLDs in 2010 were much the same as they were in 1990, with low back pain and major depressive disorder topping the list. The worldwide prevalence of back pain is 9% of adults. YLDs due to back pain increased 9% between 1990 and 2010. Overall, musculoskeletal disorders caused 21% of all YLDs. The most important were low back pain (83 million YLDs), neck pain (34 million YLDs), and osteoarthritis (17 million YLDs), with other musculoskeletal conditions contributing 28 million YLDs. Low back and neck pain contributed 70% of all YLDs from musculoskeletal disorders. Musculoskeletal disorders were important contributors to YLDs in all regions of the world. These chronic pain problems are important causes of disability.

Through its focus on disability, the GBD study has highlighted the enormous health burden imposed by non-fatal chronic conditions. It has raised the public health profile of conditions like mental health and musculoskeletal disorders that do not often cause death. The GBD study calculated disability weights between 0 (=death) and 1 (= perfect health) for 220 unique health states to capture the severity of health loss. Disability weights are calculated based on surveys of the general public. These disability weights are calculated for individuals with and without common sequelae of the index condition.

Despite the care taken by the GBD investigators to derive and validate disability weights for chronic pain conditions, Blyth and colleagues have argued that there are many reasons why the pain-related disease burden may still be underestimated:[35]

1. Case definitions for most musculoskeletal conditions have not been standardized. There are no standard International Classification of Diseases (ICD) codes for pain as a disease entity.
2. Reliable and validated self-report measures are not available for the 150 painful common musculoskeletal conditions.

3. Simple biomarkers for musculoskeletal pain are not available.
4. Pain levels and effects can fluctuate widely over the course of a musculoskeletal condition.
5. Harms associated with pain treatments (medical and surgical) are not captured in the estimation of burden.
6. Many musculoskeletal conditions do not have a specific cause or determinate course.
7. Many other health conditions have musculoskeletal pain as a component of their burden, but this may not be attributed to pain. Indeed, a substantial portion of YLDs attributed to injury, mental health and substance use disorders, and neurological conditions may be due to pain.

The 11th edition of the ICD (ICD-11) revisions that are under way may address some of these issues through reclassification of chronic primary pain and chronic musculoskeletal pain. A diagnosis of "chronic primary pain" can now be made without the need for identified biological or psychological causes of pain.[36] This change allows pain to stand on its own as a diagnosis as opposed to "chronic secondary pain," where chronic pain may be a symptom of another underlying disease.[37] *This new ICD-11 diagnosis of "chronic primary pain" is the most clear official recognition of chronic pain as a disease in its own right.*

The argument that chronic pain is itself a disease

The article that lays out the IASP argument for including the diagnosis of chronic primary pain in ICD-11 is entitled "Chronic Pain as a Symptom or a Disease."[36] This title describes the classic binary options for the status of pain within the biomedical perspective: symptom *or* disease. Bonica founded the International Association for the Study of Pain (IASP) on the idea that pain is more than a symptom, so it is not surprising that the group has endorsed classifying pain as a disease in and of itself. But the argument did not begin with these proposals for ICD-11. In his 1953 book *The Management of Pain*, Bonica distinguished normal pain (pain that functions appropriately to signal tissue damage) and abnormal pain (pain that has lost its signaling function and has become a destructive force).[10] In the 1990 edition of *The Management of Pain*, Bonica identified this abnormal pain with chronic pain, defined as pain "which persists a month beyond the usual course of an acute disease or reasonable time for an injury to heal, or pain that recurs at intervals for months or years."[38]

By 1999, Australian anesthesiologist Michael Cousins was asserting that "[c]hronic pain will be regarded as the disease of the 21st century."[39] He argued this based on the neurological changes that accompany chronic pain, producing peripheral and central sensitization of the pain system. By 2004, Siddall and Cousins expanded their argument, claiming that chronic pain had not merely become self-perpetuating, but had also become a "disease entity … having its own pathology, signs, and symptoms."[40] They advocated a "disease-based" treatment approach that addresses not only the "primary pathology" that initially caused the pain, but also the "secondary pathology" that is induced by persistent noxious inputs including peripheral and central sensitization and psychological sequelae like anxiety and catastrophizing. They even extended their recommendation to include an "environmental-based" approach that addresses "tertiary pathology" or environmental factors (biological, psychological, or social) that contribute to pain pathology.

Ted Kasin, part 3

During his clinic visit, Ted asks his doctor to obtain a magnetic resonance imaging (MRI) scan of his back "to see if something is broken back there." He explains that he has had other episodes of back pain that resolved on their own, "but this one is so bad, there must be something wrong with my spine." You explain that since he has no neurological deficits and no "red flags" for serious systemic disease like cancer, the MRI would not be useful and may just find incidental abnormalities that will lead to more tests but no benefit for him. He is not convinced. When you explain that his back pain may be due more to abnormalities in his brain than abnormalities in his back, he says, "Well, do an MRI of my brain then."

In recent years, other chronic pain investigators and clinicians have called for chronic pain to be recognized as a disease in its own right.

Daniel Clauw has argued that "fibromyalgia is a complex chronic disease that affects 3–10% of the general adult population and is principally characterized by widespread pain, and is often associated with disrupted sleep, fatigue, and comorbidities."[41] He notes other illnesses that have struggled for credibility, such as asthma and rheumatoid arthritis and other autoimmune illnesses. The strongest argument for fibromyalgia as a disease comes from the "plethora of neuroimaging" studies demonstrating brain abnormalities in fibromyalgia. Indeed, Clauw has recently extended his argument to include chronic pain more generally as "characterized by unique pathologic modifications of the central and peripheral nervous system."[42] However, he cautions that chronic pain needs to be understood within not just a biomedical model, but a broader biopsychosocial model that helps explain "variability in pain experienced by different patients with similar pain pathophysiology" through reference to an "interaction between biologic mechanisms and psychosocial factors [that] influence the interpretation of pain symptoms." Similar arguments have been made by Ohrbach concerning temporomandibular disorders,[43] Clemens and Kutch concerning pelvic pain,[44,45] and Tu concerning back pain.[46]

These arguments have been summarized by the prominent brain neuroimaging researchers Irene Tracey and Catherine Bushnell, who argue that the functional, structural, and chemical changes in the brain that are associated with chronic pain "put it into the realm of a disease state."[47] "These changes strongly support the case for dysfunctional pain processing, especially in affect regulating regions, and that these patterns of brain activity strongly reflect patients being in true discomfort and distress."[47] Tracey and Bushnell argue that their findings not only validate the status of chronic pain as a disease, but also validate the distress itself: "Chronic pain is discomforting and distressing for most patients. Providing objective proof that this is the case, in addition to listening to the patient or examining their behavior, can be obtained using functional imaging."[47]

However, we believe it is dangerous to seek to validate pain through its association with neuroimaging findings concerning blood flow (functional MRI [fMRI] scans) or radioligand uptake (positron emission tomography [PET] scans). If pain can be *validated* through association with these neuroimaging findings, it can also be *invalidated* by the lack of them. The invalidation of pain through lack of correlation with structural MRI scans of the spine or fMRI scans of the brain is not an advance for medicine. Pain is important and meaningful to people whether or not is it correlated with neuroimaging abnormalities.

A critique of chronic pain as disease

Despite its broad support within the professional pain community, there are multiple reasons to question the assertion that chronic pain is a disease. Cohen and colleagues articulated one of these succinctly in their question, "To what extent does the theory of pain-as-a-disease offer an explanation of pain?"[48] The pain-as-disease proponents cited above point to abnormalities on structural and functional neuroimaging as well as corroborating neurophysiology and neurochemistry studies to argue that there is identifiable neuropathology that causes chronic pain. The presence of this neuropathology has been found by multiple investigators using multiple methods, so it can be considered a valid finding. The problem is that pain is asserted to be *both the cause and the effect* of this neuropathology. As Cohen and colleagues state, "By asserting that pain is an agent that can cause a disease also called 'pain,' the proponents of this theory have fallen foul of circular argument." "This argument confuses pain-as-an-experience, pain-as-a-symptom, pain-as-a-pathological-entity, and pain-as-a-cause-of-pathology." It is not clear what the pain-causing and/or pain-caused neuropathology adds to the explanation of chronic pain.

Some investigators imply that the pain that causes the neuropathology is acute and nociceptive and can be linked to peripheral tissue damage, while the pain that results from the neuropathology is chronic and nociplastic (arising from altered nociceptive processing in the brain) and cannot be linked to peripheral tissue damage.[49] But this does not explain why some of the most common chronic pain syndromes like fibromyalgia and low back pain may not have an acute nociceptive phase.[50,51] Nor does it explain why the brain neuropathology associated with severe osteoarthritis of the knee reverses with successful knee replacement.[52] If the brain neuropathology is dependent upon continuous nociceptive input from the periphery, it cannot be said to be causal of the chronic pain state.

Ted Kasin, part 4

Ted's wife, Connie, drove him to your appointment and now joins you in your exam room. She hears from her husband, Ted, that he will not be getting the MRI that he wanted. She asks if her husband can do anything himself to speed his recovery from back pain. You mention that staying active is important and that walking is almost always safe with back pain. Connie says that Ted is afraid to move, for fear that he will damage his spine and end up paralyzed. You explain, based on your exam, that there are no signs that Ted's spinal cord is damaged or in danger from movement. Connie says she goes to yoga classes weekly and wonders if Ted can go. You explain that very gentle yoga would probably be OK, understanding that Ted will not be able to do all the postures that Connie can do. Connie looks enthusiastically at Ted, who just shrugs his shoulders.

Beyond these problems of circularity between changes in the brain and in the body is a more basic incoherence in the chronic-pain-as-disease argument. Pain is defined by the IASP as "an unpleasant sensory and emotional experience." But is it possible for something to be both an experience and a disease? *Is pain-as-experience identical to pain-as-disease?* This seems impossible since one is essentially subjective (as experience) while the other is essentially objective (as observable neuropathology). Or does one cause the other? In order to better understand the relation between pain-as-experience and pain-as-disease we might ask, "What are the signs and symptoms of the disease of chronic pain other than the chronic pain itself?" These might give us a path out of this vicious circularity, but they have not yet been provided.

Addiction is also not a disease

Perhaps the most important argument against chronic pain as a brain disease parallels a similar argument made against addiction as a brain disease (Table 4.1). This argument is that the disease conception of addiction or pain *leaves the patient out*. It leaves the patient, as someone capable of changes in beliefs and behaviors, out of the concept. This argument against addiction as a disease was recently summarized by Marc Lewis in the *New England Journal of*

Table 4.1 Arguments for and against disease models of addiction and chronic pain

Feature	Disease model of addiction	Disease model of chronic pain
In favor of disease model		
Functional neuroimaging abnormalities of brain	Reward processing	Sensory and emotional pain processing
Destigmatizes illness	Substance use is not a free choice or moral weakness	Pain report is not imagination or exaggeration or laziness
Therapeutic focus	Defines brain targets for therapeutic interventions	Defines brain targets for therapeutic interventions
Against disease model		
Brain (central nervous system) changes as cause or effect?	Arising from substance use or causing substance use?	Arising from pain or causing pain?
Role for learning and behavior change	No explanation for behavior changing brain, self-recovery	No explanation for behavior changing brain, self-recovery
Role of habits	Decreased drug-taking changes brain over time	Reduced catastrophizing and fear avoidance of activity decreases central sensitization
Role of context in recovery	Recover by decreasing craving or increasing salience of non-drug rewards?	Recover by decreasing pain or by increasing salience of valued physical and social activities?

Medicine.[53] As in the argument for chronic pain as a disease, the argument for addiction as a brain disease is prompted by neuroimaging findings in patients with addictions and promotion by professional organizations. This argument is advanced to destigmatize addiction by casting it as a medical problem. In the case of addiction, the argument for disease status is based on changes in reward systems wrought by exposure to drugs or alcohol rather than changes in the pain neuromatrix wrought by exposure to ongoing pain. In those with addictions (as in those with chronic pain), the brain disease model helps explain why affected persons have difficulty changing their thoughts and behaviors. Focus on these observable biological factors has helped reduce the stigma of addiction (and chronic pain) and legitimized the role of medical professionals and medications in treatment.

Alternatives to the disease model of addiction (and chronic pain) have emphasized the role of social and environmental factors that contribute to addiction. These "learning models" emphasize the important role of factors outside the boundary of the body. They also emphasize the enduring, if diminished, capacity for learning and lifestyle change that patients retain despite their addiction/chronic pain. These models can provide empowerment for patients seeking recovery and change.

Professionals have opted for the disease model of addiction over the most prominent historical alternative, which is to view addiction as a moral failure and addicts as self-indulgent and weak. Similarly, professionals have opted for the disease model of chronic pain over the most prominent historical alternative, which is to view pain as a symptom of another disease. But some patients can feel trapped in the disease model of addiction (or pain), feeling as if there is nothing they can do to "change their brain" on their own. Professionals increasingly recognize that changing behavior can change the brain itself, but many patients are not aware of this and it is not often incorporated into the disease models of addiction or pain.[54] This new model of addiction or pain as distorted learning sees it as, according to Lewis, "not just a response to stimuli but active engagement with meaningful aspects of the environment." This learning, no doubt, occurs in an altered neural and motivational environment. "Addiction neuroscientists highlight the long-lasting sensitization of the dopamine system to addictive rewards or the cues that predict them." Similarly, pain neuroscientists have highlighted the importance of the long-lasting central sensitization of nociceptive pathways and alterations in associated reward and anti-reward pathways in the process of pain becoming chronic.[55]

We do not normally think of brain pathologies as reversible through changes in thoughts and behaviors, but they might be. Lewis discusses four neurocognitive changes claimed to support the disease model of addiction:

1. The first change is a shift from impulsive drug-taking behavior mediated by the ventral striatum of the midbrain to compulsive drug-taking behavior mediated by the dorsal striatum. But all behavior becomes

more automatic as it becomes habitual. Its habitual nature does not prove an origin in brain pathology. Contingency management of addiction has shown that even entrenched compulsive behaviors can be shaped by external rewards. Similarly, chronic pain can be treated by addressing the salience of pain relief relative to other rewards rather than reducing its intensity.[56]

2. Reductions in prefrontal brain activation and synaptic density "appear to be restricted to the period of habitual drug use" and can be reversed when abstinence is learned. Brain changes can be reversed through behavioral changes. Successful treatment of chronic back pain through surgical or behavioral treatment can also reverse associated brain changes.[57]

3. The extreme or prolonged sensitization to drug-related cues in addiction can be reduced through increasing the salience and availability of non-drug rewards. Drug-taking occurs in the context of other rewards that can be strengthened. Similarly, increased commitment to values-based action can occur in the face of persistent pain.[58]

4. The desensitization to natural rewards characteristic of addiction can result from any repetitive reward-seeking behavior and is not unique to addiction. The anhedonia and anti-reward typical of chronic pain can be reversed with behavioral or pharmacological treatment.[59]

These examples suggest that brain pathologies associated with addiction and chronic pain can be reversed through changes in patients' beliefs and behaviors.

From our biomedical perspective, it is easier to conceive of brain changes (e.g., synaptic density or patterns of brain activity on MRI) as causing behavior changes than of behavior changes (e.g., drug abstinence supported through new social relationships) as causing brain changes. But neuroplasticity means that the brain changes as people learn new skills. Brain pathologies might therefore be reversible through behavior and relationship changes.

This learning perspective acknowledges and honors the fact that *most persons with addiction or with chronic pain recover without professional treatment*. Professional advice and treatment may be helpful for many patients and essential for some, *but it is not necessary for everyone*, as may be implied by the disease model. It is very difficult to quit smoking tobacco, but most who succeed do it on their own.[60] There may be considerable tension between accepting that one has a chronic disease and achieving the optimal "emphasis on motivation and self-direction" that maximizes the chance of recovery. We don't know how to combine dissimilar concepts like brain pathology and motivation, or chronic pain as brain disease and as human experience. We may be trapping patients with chronic pain into iatrogenic care-seeking by claiming they have a brain disease. If medical treatments were able to reverse or cure these brain diseases, then this disease concept would not be iatrogenic. But this is an unfulfilled promise at this time.

Conclusion: looking beyond chronic pain as disease

It is often difficult to find disease or damage that causes chronic pain. Hence, chronic pain represents an anomaly within a biomedical model that seeks the causes of subjective symptoms in objective diseases. Hence, chronic pain cannot be understood simply as a symptom. Does that mean that chronic pain is a disease? We do not think so. Although we accept that abnormalities on brain structural and functional neuroimaging are associated with chronic pain, it is not clear whether these are causes or effects of chronic pain. These brain abnormalities have not provided new targets for effective clinical treatments. And understanding chronic pain as a brain disease can exclude patients from the process of recovering from chronic pain.

However, chronic pain researchers have long sought to extend the biomedical disease model to include more psychological and social factors in their models of pathogenesis and treatment. This biopsychosocial model of chronic pain is universally endorsed by the professional pain community. We turn to consider and critique this model in our next chapter.

References

1. National Institutes of Health. What is epidemiology? 2020.
2. Skolnick P, Volkow ND. Re-energizing the development of pain therapeutics in light of the opioid epidemic. *Neuron*. 2016;92:294–297.

3. Ho JY. The contemporary American drug overdose epidemic in international perspective. *Pop Devel Rev.* 2019;45:7–40.

4. Foreman J. *A Nation in Pain.* Oxford University Press; 2014.

5. Institute of Medicine. *Relieving Pain in America: A Blue Print for Transforming Prevention, Care, Education and Research.* National Academy of Sciences; 2011.

6. Freburger JK, Holmes GM, Agans RP, et al. The rising prevalence of chronic low back pain. *Arch Intern Med.* 2009;169:251–258.

7. Sinnott P, Wagner TH. Low back pain in VA users. *Arch Intern Med.* 2009;169:1338–1339.

8. Institute of Medicine Report from the Committee on Advancing Pain Research Care and Education. *Relieving Pain in America, A Blueprint for Transforming Prevention, Care, Education and Research.* Institute of Medicine; 2011.

9. *Merriam-Webster Dictionary.* 2020.

10. Bonica J. *The Management of Pain.* Lea and Febiger; 1953.

11. Von Korff MR. Health care for chronic pain: overuse, underuse, and treatment needs. Commentary on: chronic pain and health services utilization—is there overuse of diagnostic tests and inequalities in nonpharmacologic methods utilization? *Med Care.* 2013;51:857–858.

12. Price DD. *Psychological and Neural Mechanisms of Pain.* Raven Press; 1988.

13. Campbell JN. American Pain Society 1995 Presidential Address. *Pain Forum.* 1996;5:85–88.

14. Joint Commission on Accreditation of Healthcare Organizations; National Pharmaceutical Council. *Pain: Current Understanding of Assessment, Management, and Treatments.* 2001. https://www.npcnow.org/resources/pain-current-understanding-assessment-management-and-treatments

15. Expert Committee on Cancer Pain Relief and Active Supportive Care. *Cancer Pain Relief.* World Health Organization; 1986.

16. Cassell E. *The Nature of Suffering and the Goals of Medicine.* 2nd ed. Oxford University Press; 2004.

17. Markman JD, Gewandter JS, Frazer ME. Comparison of a pain tolerability question with the numeric rating scale for assessment of self-reported chronic pain. *JAMA Netw Open.* 2020;3:e203155.

18. Adams MH, Dobscha SK, Smith NX, et al. Prevalence and correlates of low pain interference among patients with high pain intensity who are prescribed long-term opioid therapy. *J Pain.* 2018;19:1074–1081.

19. Krebs EE, Gravely A, Nugent S, et al. Effect of opioid vs. nonopioid medications on pain-related function in patients with chronic back pain or hip or knee osteoarthritis pain: The SPACE randomized clinical trial. *JAMA.* 2018;319:872–882.

20. Schumacher KL, West C, Dodd M, et al. Pain management autobiographies and reluctance to use opioids for cancer pain management. *Cancer Nurs.* 2002;25:125–133.

21. DiTomasso D. Bearing the pain: A historic review exploring the impact of science and culture on pain management for childbirth in the United States. *J Perinat Neonatal Nurs.* 2019;33:322–330.

22. Shah A, Hayes CJ, Martin BC. Characteristics of initial prescription episodes and likelihood of long-term opioid use—United States, 2006–2015. *MMWR Morb Mortal Wkly Rep.* 2017;66:265–269.

23. Sturgeon JA, Tauben D, Sullivan MD. Pain intensity as a lagging indicator of patient improvement: longitudinal relationships with sleep, mood, and function in multidisciplinary care. *J Pain.* 2019;20:S3.

24. Vinik A, Emir B, Cheung R, Whalen E. Relationship between pain relief and improvements in patient function/quality of life in patients with painful diabetic peripheral neuropathy or postherpetic neuralgia treated with pregabalin. *Clin Ther.* 2013;35:612–623.

25. Vinik A, Emir B, Parsons B, Cheung R. Prediction of pregabalin-mediated pain response by severity of sleep disturbance in patients with painful diabetic neuropathy and post-herpetic neuralgia. *Pain Med.* 2014;15:661–670.

26. Rej S, Dew MA, Karp JF. Treating concurrent chronic low back pain and depression with low-dose venlafaxine: an initial identification of "easy-to-use" clinical predictors of early response. *Pain Med.* 2014;15:1154–62.

27. Kamper SJ, Apeldoorn AT, Chiarotto A, et al. Multidisciplinary biopsychosocial rehabilitation for chronic low back pain. *Cochrane Database Syst Rev.* 2014;9:CD000963.

28. Lynch-Jordan AM, Sil S, Peugh J, et al. Differential changes in functional disability and pain intensity over the course of psychological treatment for children with chronic pain. *Pain.* 2014;155:1955–61.

29. Williams ACC FE, Hearn L, Eccleston C. Psychological therapies for the management of chronic pain (excluding headache) in adults. *Cochrane Database Syst Rev.* 2020;8:CD007407.

30. *National Pain Strategy: A Comprehensive Population Health-Level Strategy for Pain.* 2016.

31. Dahlhamer J, Lucas J, Zelaya C, et al. Prevalence of chronic pain and high-impact chronic pain among adults—United States, 2016. *MMWR Morb Mortal Wkly Rep.* 2018;67:1001–1006.

32. Von Korff M, DeBar LL, Krebs EE, et al. Graded chronic pain scale revised: mild, bothersome, and high-impact chronic pain. *Pain.* 2020;161:651–661.

33. Murray C, Lopez A, eds. *The Global Burden of Disease: A Comprehensive Assessment of Mortality and Disability from Diseases, Injuries, and Risk Factors in 1990 and Projected to 2020.* Harvard University Press; 1996.

34. Vos T, Flaxman AD, Naghavi M, et al. Years lived with disability (YLDs) for 1160 sequelae of 289 diseases and injuries 1990-2010: a systematic analysis for the Global Burden of Disease Study 2010. *Lancet.* 2012;380:2163–96.

35. Blyth FM, Briggs AM, Schneider CH, et al. The global burden of musculoskeletal pain: where to from here? *Am J Public Health.* 2019;109:35–40.

36. Nicholas M, Vlaeyen JWS, Rief W, et al. The IASP classification of chronic pain for ICD-11: chronic primary pain. *Pain.* 2019;160:28–37.

37. Treede RD, Rief W, Barke A, et al. Chronic pain as a symptom or a disease: the IASP Classification of Chronic Pain for the International Classification of Diseases (ICD-11). *Pain.* 2019;160:19–27.

38. Bonica J. *The Management of Pain.* Lea & Febiger; 1990.

39. Cousins MJ. Pain: the past, present, and future of anesthesiology? The E. A. Rovenstine Memorial Lecture. *Anesthesiology.* 1999;91:538–551.

40. Siddall PJ, Cousins MJ. Persistent pain as a disease entity: implications for clinical management. *Anesth Analg.* 2004;99:510–520.

41. Clauw DJ, D'Arcy Y, Gebke K, et al. Normalizing fibromyalgia as a chronic illness. *Postgrad Med.* 2018;130:9–18.

42. Clauw DJ, Essex MN, Pitman V, Jones KD. Reframing chronic pain as a disease, not a symptom: rationale and implications for pain management. *Postgrad Med.* 2019;131:185–198.

43. Ohrbach R, Dworkin SF. The evolution of TMD diagnosis: past, present, future. *J Dent Res.* 2016;95:1093–1101.

44. Clemens JQ, Mullins C, Ackerman AL, et al. Urologic chronic pelvic pain syndrome: insights from the MAPP Research Network. *Nat Rev Urol.* 2019;16:187–200.

45. Kutch JJ, Ichesco E, Hampson JP, et al. Brain signature and functional impact of centralized pain: a multidisciplinary approach to the study of chronic pelvic pain (MAPP) network study. *Pain.* 2017;158(10):1979–1991.

46. Tu Y, Jung M, Gollub RL, et al. Abnormal medial prefrontal cortex functional connectivity and its association with clinical symptoms in chronic low back pain. *Pain.* 2019;160:1308–1318.

47. Tracey I, Bushnell MC. How neuroimaging studies have challenged us to rethink: is chronic pain a disease? *J Pain.* 2009;10:1113–1120.

48. Cohen M, Quintner J, Buchanan D. Is chronic pain a disease? *Pain Med.* 2013;14:1284–1288.

49. Heinricher MM. Pain modulation and the transition from acute to chronic pain. *Adv Exp Med Biol*. 2016;904:105–115.

50. Buskila D, Neumann L. Musculoskeletal injury as a trigger for fibromyalgia/ posttraumatic fibromyalgia. *Curr Rheumatol Rep*. 2000;2:104–108.

51. Hadler NM, Tait RC, Chibnall JT. Back pain in the workplace. *JAMA*. 2007;297:1594–1596.

52. Rodriguez-Raecke R, Niemeier A, et al. Structural brain changes in chronic pain reflect probably neither damage nor atrophy. *PLoS One*. 2013;8:e54475.

53. Lewis M. Brain change in addiction as learning, not disease. *N Engl J Med*. 2018;379:1551–1560.

54. Doidge N. *The Brain That Changes Itself*. Viking Press; 2007.

55. Borsook D, Youssef AM, Simons L, et al. When pain gets stuck: the evolution of pain chronification and treatment resistance. *Pain*. 2018;159(12):2421–2436.

56. Sullivan MD, Vowles KE. Patient action: as means and end for chronic pain care. *Pain*. 2017;158:1405–7.

57. Seminowicz DA, Wideman TH, Naso L, et al. Effective treatment of chronic low back pain in humans reverses abnormal brain anatomy and function. *J Neurosci*. 2011;18:7540–7550.

58. Vilardaga R, Sullivan MD, Davies PD, Vowles K. Theoretical grounds of pain tracker self manager: An acceptance and commitment therapy digital intervention for patients with chronic pain. *J Contextual Behav Sci*. 2020;15:172–180.

59. Elman I, Borsook D. Threat response system: parallel brain processes in pain vis-à-vis fear and anxiety. *Front Psychiatry*. 2018;9:29.

60. Stead LF, Buitrago D, Preciado N, et al. Physician advice for smoking cessation. *Cochrane Database Syst Rev*. 2013;5:CD000165.

5
Looking beyond a biopsychosocial model of pain

> If you are distressed by anything external, the pain is not due to the thing itself, but to your estimate of it; and this you have the power to revoke at any moment.
>
> Marcus Aurelius, *Meditations*

These days, there is universal endorsement of a biopsychosocial (BPS) model of chronic pain. This model is defined by *Merriam-Webster* as "of, relating to, or concerned with the biological, psychological, and social aspects in contrast to the strictly biomedical aspects of disease."[1] The 2011 Institute of Medicine (IOM) report contains this typical passage: "Numerous factors—involving the type of pain, one's background and personal traits, and the family and social environments—affect an individual's treatment plan."[2] The 2016 National Pain Strategy contains similar statements: "Chronic pain is a biopsychosocial condition that often requires integrated, multi-modal, and interdisciplinary treatment, all components of which should be evidence-based." These models seem so comprehensive, encompassing everything from molecules to cultures, it is hard to imagine that anything relevant has been omitted. But it is important to understand that the biological, the psychological, and the social factors incorporated into the BPS model are not treated equally in the ways that the model is usually conceptualized and implemented.

In an exhaustive 2007 review of the BPS model of pain, Gatchel and colleagues claim:

> The biopsychosocial model focuses on both disease and illness, with illness being viewed as the complex interaction of biological, psychological,

and social factors.... [D]*isease* is defined as an objective biological event involving the disruption of specific body structures or organ systems caused by either anatomical, pathological, or physiological changes. In contrast, *illness* refers to a subjective experience or self-attribution that a disease is present.... The distinction between disease and illness is analogous to the distinction that can be made between *nociception* and *pain*.[3(p599)]

According to this review, the BPS model addresses the translation of objective disease into experienced illness, or nociception into pain (Figure 5.1).

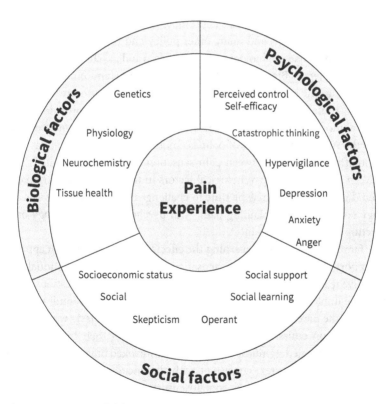

Figure 5.1. BPS model diagram

Reprinted from: Adams LM, Turk DC. Central sensitization and the biopsychosocial approach to understanding pain. *J Appl Behav Res.* 2018; 23:e12125. https://doi.org/10.1111/jabr.12125.

The BPS model has supported an interdisciplinary model of care that integrates multiple disciplines (physician, psychologist, physical therapist, nurse, and others) into the care of the patient with chronic pain. It reaches beyond a purely biomedical approach to chronic pain.[4] The BPS model thus addresses a diverse set of influences on chronic pain, but it doesn't question the independence of the "objective biological event" of disease. This primacy granted to biology is an important and often neglected limitation of the BPS model.

Pain as a sensation that prompts an emotional reaction

The biopsychosocial model that is promoted in the IOM pain report, the National Pain Strategy, and many other policy and research reports about chronic pain focuses on biological *causes* of pain and psychosocial *modifiers* of that experience. Biological factors are allowed to stand on their own as causes of chronic pain, while psychological and social factors are not. There are many roots for this biocentric thinking. Since Descartes provided a mechanical model for pain production within the body, we have moved away from the Aristotelean model of pain as emotion to a model of pain as sensation. The distinction between pain sensation and emotion parallels that between biological and psychological factors in that pain sensation is considered primary. But it may be time to challenge the standard view that biology comes first in explaining pain, with psychology and sociology only affecting the reaction to pain.

A famous 1999 study concerning the effects of hypnosis on pain appears to support the idea that pain is a sensation that provokes an emotional and cognitive reaction. Rainville and colleagues used hypnotic suggestions to reduce the unpleasantness of the pain produced by noxious stimuli without changing the perceived intensity. This occurred while subjects were undergoing positron emission tomography (PET) scans of their brain activity. These scans revealed significant changes in pain-evoked brain activity within anterior cingulate cortex, consistent with the encoding of perceived unpleasantness, whereas primary somatosensory cortex activation was unaltered.[5] This was followed by another experiment using hypnosis in normal subjects to alter the experience of experimental heat pain. Hypnotic suggestions directed at reducing pain unpleasantness did reduce experienced unpleasantness but not pain intensity. On the other hand, hypnotic suggestions directed at reducing pain intensity reduced both intensity and unpleasantness. These experiments were interpreted as showing that perception of pain intensity was separate and prior to perception of pain unpleasantness.[6] It is not clear whether these findings concerning acute experimental pain apply to chronic pain. Some studies reviewed later suggest they do not.

These acute pain experimental findings concerning the sequential relation between sensory and emotional aspects of pain perception have been reflected in the primary behavioral therapy used to treat patients with chronic pain, cognitive–behavioral therapy (CBT). CBT has become the dominant application of the BPS model in the treatment of chronic pain. It grew out of the operant behavioral therapy for chronic pain developed by Fordyce that sought to shape pain behavior (like resting and limping and asking for help) and thereby reduce disability and suffering associated with chronic pain. CBT added cognitive techniques addressing distorted cognitions like catastrophizing and fear avoidance, as well as coping skills training like pacing and relaxation skills. But its goal remained living well with chronic pain rather than reducing or eliminating this pain. Recently, Moseley and Butler argued that the CBT approach is "more consistent with 'pain is unavoidable—suffering is optional.' That is, CBT aims to manage pain, rather than to treat it."[7(p810)] In the standard CBT model, pain is given to the person, but suffering is constructed by the person. This model has predecessors in both the East (e.g., Buddhism) and the West (e.g., Stoicism), but may not be consistent with the most recent pain neuroscience that considers both pain and suffering to be constructed by a brain aimed at survival.

This CBT approach is consistent with a version of the BPS model that looks at biological factors as the primary causes of pain and psychological and social factors as modifiers of that causal process, but not independent causes themselves. One of the pioneers of the CBT approach, Dennis Turk, states in an early review paper:

> The cognitive-behavioral (CB) perspective is concerned both with helping with residual pain after (medical) treatment and with identifying and treating some of the factors that may interact with physical pathology to maintain and potentiate pain and disability. People respond to medical conditions based in part on their beliefs about illness and their symptoms.[8(p575)]

Thus the CBT approach concerns someone's *response* to a medical condition rather than the *cause* of the medical condition itself. From the same article:

> Behavior and emotions are influenced by interpretations of events, rather than solely by objective characteristics. Thus pain, when interpreted as signifying ongoing tissue damage, a progressive disease, or for which there is no known cause, is likely to produce considerably more suffering and behavioral dysfunction than if it is viewed as being the result of a known cause that is expected to improve.[8(p577)]

CBT thus addresses the *interpretation* of pain and the behavior and emotions that accompany pain rather than the *causation* of pain itself. It aims to reduce the impact of pain by focusing on psychosocial modifiers of that pain rather than the pain itself. In this way CBT and pain psychology have carved out a space in the clinical world of chronic pain care as a *supplement* to the biomedical approach rather than as a *replacement* for it. CBT has been proven efficacious for chronic pain management in many controlled trials, but the effect sizes produced by CBT have generally been small.[9]

CBT has been successfully used to help patients manage pain of clear medical origin as well as pain of unclear origin. During the early years of pre-CBT pain psychology (1960s–1970s), psychological treatment was thought by many patients and physicians as appropriate *only* for pain of psychological origin.[10] Recent CBT literature rarely addresses the psychological or social causation of pain directly. But during the earlier phase of operant behavioral treatment of chronic pain, the possibility of psychogenic pain was directly dismissed. Bill Fordyce, one of the originators of pain psychology and operant treatment of chronic pain, railed against the idea that psychopathology could be brought in to explain pain that physical tissue pathology could not explain: "There is something wrong with the body or, failing that, the problem is with his or her mind. If physical findings are lacking, the pain problem becomes psychogenic or such variants thereof as somatization, conversion reaction, hypochondriasis, etc."[11(p115)] At this time (1970s–1980s), the reigning theories of psychogenic pain were psychoanalytic. But these theories were seen by many patients, and by Fordyce, as denying the reality of the patient's pain: "When that (psychogenic) assumption is made, the clinician often thinks of the patient's pain as not real. or as exaggerated or malingered. The implication is that the patient is not really suffering. Overall, the effect of this approach is to the victim."[11(p117)] Fordyce, Turk, and the bulk of CBT therapists therefore carefully avoid talk about psychosocial *causes* of pain in favor of speaking about psychosocial *modifiers* of biological causation. The notion of psychogenic pain is not part of the BPS model used in current chronic pain care.

Not all chronic pain experts find this interpretation of the BPS model to be adequate. In a 2014 article, Carr and Bradshaw proposed

> to reframe the pain curriculum from its current standard formulation as a bottom-up "biopsychosocial" phenomenon to a top-down "sociopsychobiological" one. We believe that "hard" scientific evidence supporting the reframing of pain as an interpersonal, inherently social process has accumulated to reach a tipping point such that relatively little effort will be needed to implement this change.[12(p12)]

They lament that much more emphasis is placed on biological mechanisms of pain at the molecular and cellular level than on "intersubjective processes including empathy, social bonding and isolation-induced suffering." They argue that "a dysphoric social dimension involving isolation, withdrawal, and distress and often stigma contributes to the multidimensional experience of pain nearly as much as nociception." We ignore everyday evidence of a mother's ability to soothe her toddler in favor of an emphasis on mechanism-based pain therapy. The reductionist program that explains bigger parts and processes in terms of smaller parts and processes has been very successful in medicine over the past two centuries. But bringing chronic pain as disease within this reductionist story of molecules and cells minimizes the importance of personal and interpersonal causes and remedies for human pain.

Ted Kasin, part 1

Ted and his wife, Connie (from Chapter 4), return for a follow-up appointment a month after their previous visit. Ted has been on a few walks around the block with Connie and her dog, Bubbles. This did not worsen Ted's pain, but it did not make it any better either. Connie has tried to get

Ted to come to yoga, but Ted is still scared and not eager to go to a class "full of women in yoga pants." Connie jokes, "Hey, those are my friends!" Ted responds glumly, "It must be nice to have friends." Connie explains that Ted had good pals on the auto assembly line. They stayed in touch when they were laid off, but now the rest have gone back to work and he does not hear from them. "He feels like he has lost his friends as well as his back," Connie explains. "His social life just disappeared."

What would a sociopsychobiological pain model look like?

Human pain and suffering have many origins. But in the modern era, we have tried to isolate pain as a medical problem from the rest of human suffering. Our medical perspective gives privilege to pain caused by changes inside the body, so we dismiss pain caused by changes outside the body as non-medical, as just psychological or social issues. These are personal concerns, not medical concerns. Though clinicians rarely say it explicitly, patients hear these dismissals as "your pain is all in your head." This dismissal implies that the pain is not only psychological but also imaginary or exaggerated, and that the appropriate response is to "just get over it." Professional medicine has embraced pain as a medical problem, but only partially. It wants pain to have a clear medical cause, meaning some objective disease or injury.

Epidemiology investigates not only the prevalence of chronic pain, but also its associations and its origins. However, it does not look everywhere equally for these associations and origins. Epidemiology serves pathophysiology in our modern explanation of disease, so it looks for those associations that can be most readily translated into pathophysiological mechanisms that can be addressed and treated in the clinical setting.[13]

Consider the case of low back pain. Up to 84% of adults may have an episode of back pain in their lifetimes, with 26% reporting at least a full day of back pain in the past 3 months.[14] As McGuirk and Bogduk report in the latest edition of *Bonica's Management of Pain*, "Although the possible sources of back pain have been demonstrated [through experimental stimulation studies], its causes [in clinical practice] have been more elusive. Conventional methods of assessment and investigation typically fail to identify the cause of chronic low back pain in the majority of patients."[15(p375)] They go on to explain that "many conditions traditionally considered to be possible causes of chronic low back pain *are actually not causes*." Degenerative changes in the back are common, but they are also common in persons with no back pain. Tumors and infections can cause back pain, but they are rare. Back pain is often attributed to "muscle sprain, ligament sprain, segmental dysfunction, and trigger points," but these are difficult to verify and it is unclear how they can cause pain to be chronic. Dysfunction of sacroiliac and facet joints can produce pain that can be blocked with nerve blocks, but this blocking rarely lasts very long. Herniated intervertebral lumbar disks can cause back pain and sciatic nerve pain, but they are also seen in persons with no back pain. Surgery can speed recovery of sciatica, but without surgery pain decreases in approximately 87% of patients within 3 months.[16(pp1105–1122)] Thus the discovery of causes that would allow us to base therapy on the pathophysiological mechanisms of back pain has been elusive.

If we look at the risk factors for developing low back pain, especially chronic low back pain, a much broader set of issues is relevant. Physical factors such as older age, female gender, obesity, and smoking are important. But so are psychological factors (anxiety, depression), social factors (low education, life stress), and occupational factors (physically or psychologically strenuous work, sedentary work, low social support, job dissatisfaction).[14] A recent review of the social determinants of low back pain synthesized 41 studies with data from over 2 million adults in 17 countries. Strong evidence for independent social effects was found, including place of residence, race, occupation, gender, education, socioeconomic status, and social capital.[17] Education and socioeconomic status showed the strongest effects. But many of these risks are difficult to treat in the clinical setting, and it is challenging to study them in experimental studies or controlled clinical trials. Because the mechanisms of these effects are elusive, we have been hampered in developing a comprehensive sociopsychobiological model of back pain.

Could a deeper and more pervasive bias in our thinking about causes of back pain be guiding our attention here? Consider one of the largest prospective studies of chronic pain in the world. The World Health Organization (WHO)'s Collaborative Study of Psychological Problems in General Health Care screened nearly 26,000 primary care patients and interviewed nearly 5500 across 15 centers in 14 countries around the world. Across all the centers, 22% of patients had persistent pain, though prevalence varied between 5% and 33%. Those with persistent pain were more than four times as likely to have an anxiety or depressive disorder than those without. This relationship between pain and distress was more consistent across countries than the relationship between pain and disability.[18] Approximately 3200 patients were interviewed 12 months after their initial interview. Of those with pain at baseline, about half had not recovered and 9% had new persistent pain. Of note, "A persistent pain disorder at baseline predicted the onset of a psychological disorder to the same degree that a baseline psychological disorder predicted the subsequent onset of persistent pain."[(p149)] The authors concluded, "We found a strong and symmetrical relationship between persistent pain and psychological disorder. Impairment of daily activities appears to be a central component of that relationship." Anxiety and depression are not simply a "reasonable response" to chronic pain, but can be causes that precede it.

The WHO study, and other careful longitudinal studies, have documented a bidirectional, even symmetrical, relationship between chronic pain disorders and anxiety or depressive disorders. These anxiety and depressive disorders not only are associated with greater pain severity, worse functioning, more disability, and greater costs of care in patients who have them in addition to chronic pain,[19] but they also often *precede* the chronic pain problem.[20-22] *Suffering causes chronic pain as often as chronic pain causes suffering.* These findings have been ignored or dismissed because they do not fit into the dominant scientific and moral image of pain in our culture, which sees pain as physically caused or having no real cause at all.

Psychogenic pain: old and new

In modern medicine, the concept of psychogenic pain is poorly defined and is simply opposed to "real pain" or pain that can be associated with observable tissue damage in the body. Here, psychogenic pain is implied to be "unreal" or "imaginary" pain, though no one ever explains what that is. Do patients ever complain of unreal or imaginary pain? In the most sophisticated contexts, psychogenic pain is opposed to "somatogenic pain"—that is, purely physical or physiological pain produced by the body and brain, without any involvement of psychological processes.

Philosophers have been fascinated by this purely physical form of pain since Descartes proposed his mechanical model of pain perception. He illustrated this model with the famous image of the boy with his foot in the fire (see Figure 1.3 in Chapter 1). The damage produced by the fire tugged on a nerve that ran from the boy's foot, through his spinal cord, and up into his brain where pain was produced, much like someone ringing a church bell. In the 1970s and 1980s, materialist philosophers boldly predicted that we would soon stop expressing pain through terms like "ouch!" that referred to the subjective experience of pain and would replace these antiquated folk psychology concepts with modern scientific descriptions of the objective physiological processes that produce pain such as "my c-fibers are firing." Unfortunately for these philosophers, it turns out that activation of c-fibers by peripheral nociceptors is neither necessary nor sufficient for the experience of pain.

But the dream of finding a purely objective "neurological signature" for pain lives on. In 2013, the *New England Journal of Medicine* published an article entitled "An fMRI-Based Neurologic Signature of Physical Pain" by Wager and colleagues.[23] This paper described a pattern of brain activation (as indicated by differences in blood flow) produced by experimental heat stimuli that predicted experienced pain intensity in individual persons with high sensitivity and specificity. The title of this paper makes its agenda clear: It is describing a *neurological* signature of *physical* pain. There is no room here for subjectivity or psychological processes. The authors argue that this purely objective access to pain will allow us to bypass the flawed and mediated access to pain provided by patient self-report. This idea of a fully objectified and de-psychologized pain is the concept against which psychogenic pain is now generally defined. But this is a trap: Only when we escape the dualistic opposition between purely psychogenic and purely somatogenic pain will we achieve a clinically useful and philosophically robust concept of pain.

History of psychogenic pain concepts

The recent history of the psychiatric diagnosis of "psychogenic pain" illustrates the problems of the dualistic framework. Before 1980, psychologically caused pain was understood in terms of psychodynamic processes. Sigmund

Freud drew upon the work of Anton Mesmer and Jean Charcot that showed hypnosis could reverse paralysis and other conversion symptoms. Freud interpreted these effects of hypnosis as evidence that powerful unconscious processes could cause physical symptoms like pain. In a famous 1959 paper, "Psychogenic Pain and the Pain-Prone Patient," George Engel proposed that psychogenic pain arose from guilt and an intolerance of success.[24] He argued that pain functioned as a substitute for loss or a replacement for aggression. In the 1968 second edition of the American Psychiatric Association's *Diagnostic and Statistical Manual* (DSM-II), psychogenic pain was codified as part of psychophysiological disorders and described under "painful conditions caused by emotional factors."[25]

In 1980, DSM-III introduced a new diagnostic category for pain problems, "psychogenic pain disorder."[26] To qualify for this diagnosis, a patient needed to have severe and prolonged pain inconsistent with neuroanatomical distribution of pain receptors or without detectable organic etiology or pathophysiologic mechanism. Difficulties in establishing that pain was psychogenic led to changes in the diagnosis for DSM-III-R, published in 1987.[27] Here, the diagnosis was renamed "somatoform pain disorder," and requirements for etiological psychological factors and lack of other contributing mental disorders were eliminated and a requirement for "preoccupation with pain for at least six months" was added. In DSM-III-R, therefore, somatoform pain disorder *becomes purely a diagnosis of exclusion.* The diagnosis is made when medical disorders are excluded in a patient "preoccupied" with pain. The search for positive signs of psychological causation of pain is abandoned.

When it came time to revise these criteria for DSM-IV in 1994, the subcommittee on pain disorders found that, despite these changes, "somatoform pain disorder" was rarely used in research projects or clinical practice. They identified a number of reasons for this, including (1) the meaning of "preoccupation with pain" is unclear, (2) whether pain exceeds that expected on the basis of tissue damage is difficult to determine, and (3) the term "somatoform pain disorder" implies that this pain is somehow different from organic pain. This spelled the end of "somatoform pain disorder." Psychogenic pain survived in DSM-IV as a subtype of the psychiatric diagnosis of pain disorder.[28] Though great efforts were made to overcome the shortcomings of the DSM-III and DSM-III-R definitions, in DSM-IV pain disorder remained a diagnosis of exclusion founded upon unclear notions of medically unexplained pain and psychologically caused pain.[29]

The current 2013 edition of the DSM (DSM-5)[30] does not include a pain-specific disorder. Instead, it includes somatic symptom disorder (SSD), a single diagnosis that replaces three of the DSM-IV somatoform disorders (somatization disorder, pain disorder, and undifferentiated somatoform disorder). The diagnostic criteria for SSD require the presence of one or more physical symptoms lasting 6 months or longer that are associated with excessive thoughts, feelings, or behaviors. The diagnosis of somatic symptom disorder in DSM-5 thus abandons criteria requiring that pain be medically unexplained or psychologically caused in favor of a focus on excessive concern. But critics have argued that this makes the diagnosis far too inclusive and risks mislabeling medical illness as mental disorder.[31-33] These critics propose reintroducing the former criteria concerning medical and psychological causation.

How are we to escape this oscillation between psychogenic pain definitions that invoke mysterious psychological causes and those that only note the absence of clear medical causes? We will advance only by grasping that the debate is trapped in a dualistic opposition of physical and psychological causes. As Fordyce argued, we are drawn to the concept of psychogenic pain because it fills the gaps left when our attempts to explain clinical pain exclusively in terms of tissue pathology and nociception fail. But the concept of psychogenic pain, as it has been laid out in recent editions of the DSM, is an empty concept. Positive criteria for the identification of psychogenic pain, mechanisms for the production of psychogenic pain, and specific therapies for psychogenic pain are lacking.[34] This is because we are trying to define a gap or a hole in our current means of pain explanation by tissue damage. Is it surprising that this gap has no definable shape? The diagnosis of many psychiatric disorders, such as depression and posttraumatic stress disorder (PTSD), can be very helpful to clinicians caring for patients with chronic pain by pointing toward specific effective therapies. But the diagnosis of psychogenic pain on the basis of the absence of identifiable medical causes too often only serves to stigmatize further the patient who experiences chronic pain. An injured worker who is diagnosed with somatic symptom disorder gets little guidance about how to get better, but may lose his workers' compensation benefits.

Ted Kasin, part 2

Ted returns to the clinic with Connie. She says that he has been to yoga with her, but only once. While Ted was trying to get into a posture, the yoga teacher put his hands on Ted to gently correct his form and Ted freaked out. He was startled, jumped up and hurt his back, and then limped out of class. Ted explains that he just doesn't like to be touched without warning. Connie confirms that, when they were first dating, he became comfortable with her touching him only very gradually: "He is very jumpy, always has been." When you ask if this has been true for Ted's whole life, Ted shrugs, "I guess." Connie looks over to Ted for permission, then tells you that Ted's father used to beat him. "It started out as spanking when he was little, but then progressed to punching when Ted was a teen-ager. Once, after Ted took the car out without permission, he was hit in the back with a 2-by-4. He still has nightmares about that sometimes."

Role of psychological trauma in chronic pain

Exposure to events that pose a serious threat to personal and bodily integrity can be psychologically traumatic. It is estimated that 70% of adults living in the United States have been exposed to significant traumatic events.[35,36] Most people who experience traumatic events do not experience lasting effects, though people exposed to motor vehicle accidents, sexual assault, and military combat appear more likely to have lasting effects of trauma. The most-studied psychological effect of psychological trauma is PTSD. The lifetime prevalence of PTSD in the U.S. population is 7.8%. PTSD symptoms emerge in 30% of those exposed to extreme stressors within days of the exposure, but usually resolve in a few weeks. For 10% to 20% of those exposed, PTSD symptoms persist beyond 6 months with impairment in functioning. Of patients with PTSD, 50% improve without treatment in 1 year, while a third develop a chronic disorder that lasts for years.[37] Hence, most persons heal spontaneously from even significant psychological trauma.

PTSD is defined in DSM-5 as having seven components:

1. Exposure to severe trauma, such as threatened death

2. Re-experiencing of the traumatic event through intrusive memories, nightmares, or flashbacks
3. Avoidance of trauma reminders
4. Negative alterations in cognition and mood such as inability to remember traumatic event as well as negative beliefs and emotions regarding the event
5. Altered arousal and reactivity such as irritable or self-destructive behavior
6. Persistence for over 1 month
7. Significant distress or functional impairment.[30]

Physical trauma may be one component of the psychological trauma, but need not be.

There are many other effects of psychological trauma besides PTSD, as documented in the Adverse Childhood Experiences (ACE) study of the U.S. Centers for Disease Control and Prevention. The ACE study studied eight serious adverse childhood experiences (e.g., abuse, neglect, witnessed violence) in 17,337 adult health maintenance organization (HMO) members. The documented effects of these experiences include not only mental illness and substance abuse, but also obesity, insomnia, promiscuity, violence, and multiple somatic symptoms, including pain.[38] Those with four or more ACEs were more likely to use prescription medications, including psychotropic medications.[39] The results of trauma, especially childhood trauma, thus reach far beyond PTSD, but PTSD is our best available marker to track the effects of trauma in adult populations.

Chronic pain is reported by 35% to 50% of patients with PTSD, regardless of the trauma experienced.[40] The most common kinds of pain are pelvic pain, low back pain, facial pain, bladder pain, and fibromyalgia. PTSD is also common among patients presenting for care of chronic pain, with 7% to 50% meeting criteria.[41] PTSD is especially prevalent in some subsets of the population with chronic pain. It is seen in 39% of motor vehicle accident survivors who present for care of pain, as well as 39% of assault victims and 35% of injured workers sent for rehabilitation. Among patients with fibromyalgia, 20% currently meet criteria for PTSD, while 42% have met criteria at some point in their life. In young adults, PTSD is the psychiatric disorder most strongly associated with medically unexplained pain.[42]

PTSD and chronic pain may reinforce each other in multiple ways. Severe acute pain can be traumatic. Acute pain level after trauma predicts PTSD.[43] Chronic pain may function as a reminder of the trauma, setting up a cycle of mutual maintenance between pain and PTSD. PTSD also prompts the re-experiencing of trauma, which itself triggers arousal that leads to avoidance and pain through muscle tension. This can lead to perpetual avoidance. In a 2010 prospective study, baseline re-experiencing and avoidance predicted arousal and pain at 3 months, which then predicted re-experiencing, avoidance, arousal and pain at 12 months.[44] If the original injury is seen as the result of injustice or unfair treatment, both PTSD and pain are likely to persist.[45]

PTSD is not only common in patients with chronic pain, but it also changes the experience of chronic pain and the recommended treatment. Chronic pain patients who have PTSD report more intense pain and affective distress as well as higher levels of disability than those without PTSD. In a landmark study of 141,029 Iraq/Afghanistan veterans with chronic pain treated in Veterans Affairs hospitals, it was noted that approximately 10% received opioid therapy (e.g., morphine, oxycodone). This included 6% of veterans without mental health disorders, 12% with non-PTSD mental health disorders, and 18% of veterans with PTSD. Thus, mental health disorders doubled the rate of opioid therapy and PTSD tripled the rate of opioid therapy compared to veterans without mental health disorders. Furthermore, veterans with PTSD were more likely to receive higher-dose opioids, two or more opioids, concurrent sedative–hypnotics, and early opioid refills. They also showed the highest rates of adverse clinical outcomes from opioid therapy.[46]

This PTSD research suggests that psychological trauma may play as important a role as physical trauma in the development, severity, course, and treatment of chronic pain, and in the prescription and outcome of opioid therapy. Indeed, in a sample of 1206 patients seen at the University of Washington Center for Pain Relief, endorsement of zero to four PTSD symptom domains was linearly related to the severity of all pain clinical outcomes monitored, including not only depression and anxiety, but also pain intensity, activity interference, sleep interference, disability, overall health status, and opioid risk.[47]

Other research suggests that the importance of physical and psychological factors in the causation of chronic pain may shift over time. The sequential understanding of pain's sensory and affective aspects, indebted to Rainville's previously discussed hypnosis experiments and other studies, may not apply to chronic pain. A prospective study of patients with low back pain using multiple functional magnetic resonance imaging (fMRI) brain scans showed that as back pain evolves from acute and subacute to chronic, the associated brain activity shifts from nociceptive regions involved in acute pain to emotion-related circuitry.[48] Importantly, this back pain usually feels the same to the patient when it is acute (less than 3 months' duration) and when it is chronic (over 3 months' duration). Thus, the brain is involved in both acute back pain that we are likely to label somatogenic due to its frequent association with physical trauma, and in chronic back pain that we are likely to label psychogenic due to our inability to identify any associated damage to the back. Hence, our opposition of somatogenic and psychogenic pain may be based on outdated neuroscience and not clinically useful.

Medical clinicians are not only inclined to distinguish pain with physical causes from pain with psychological causes; as clinicians embedded in the biomedical environment, we are also inclined to dismiss psychogenic pain as less real and less important than somatogenic pain. This is most apparent in medicolegal contexts where psychological trauma is much more difficult to verify and much less likely to result in compensation in tort or workers' injury cases.[49] But it is also true in many clinical situations where pain with a localized bodily cause is considered not only more verifiable, but also more responsive to medical interventions. However, physical pain and social pain may be more similar than we think.

Physical and social pain arise from similar neurophysiological processes

Most people would rather have a broken leg than a broken heart. We experience social rejection, exclusion, or loss as among the most aversive experiences that we endure. Research, initially out of the laboratory of Naomi Eisenberger at the University of California at Los Angeles, suggests that painful feelings produced by social disconnection activate the same brain centers as experiences of physical pain. She has shown that subjects who suffer social exclusion during a virtual game show patterns of brain activation on fMRI (e.g., in the anterior cingulate cortex and the anterior insula) that are very similar to the patterns of activation induced by physical noxious

stimuli and are proportional to the feelings of exclusion.[50] She has hypothe-
sized that "threats to social connection may be just as detrimental to survival
as threats to basic physical safety and thus may be processed by some of the
same underlying neural circuitry."[51(p430)] She suggests that in social primates
"the social attachment system may have piggybacked onto the opioid sub-
strates of the physical pain system to maintain proximity with others, elic-
iting distress upon separation (through low opioid receptor activity) and
comfort upon reunion (through high opioid receptor activity)."[(p431)]

Other research supports this parallel between social and physical
pain, from damage to social relationships and damage to bodily tissue.
Sensitivity to social and physical pain tend to vary together. In clinical
studies, patients with chronic pain are more sensitive to social pain, as evi-
denced by greater fear and avoidance of social interactions.[52] Conversely,
heightened sensitivity to social pain (e.g., anxious attachment style) is associated with more physical symptoms, including pain.[53] In experimental
studies, individuals who are more sensitive to physical noxious stimuli
also report more social pain in response to social exclusion.[54] Finally,
social pain and physical pain respond to the same treatments. It is well
known that opioids relieve social pain as well as physical pain.[55] It is perhaps more surprising that the over-the-counter physical pain reliever acetaminophen (Tylenol) was shown to reduce social pain in a double-blind
placebo-controlled study.[56]

Recent research suggests that the boundaries between somatogenic and
psychogenic pain are not as clear as traditionally claimed. Central sensitization leading to enhanced pain sensitivity was originally attributed to an
ongoing injury-induced nociceptive barrage of the central nervous system.[57]
But there is strong evidence that patients with chronic pain who have evidence of central sensitization (including generalized pain) also have higher
rates of anxiety and depression and higher rates of psychological trauma.[58]
Patients with low back pain with catastrophic cognitions (e.g., pain is inescapable or overwhelming) also have signs of central sensitization such as
increased temporal summation and decreased conditioned pain modulation on sensory testing.[59] Both trauma exposure and PTSD symptoms have
been shown to be related to multiple measures of central sensitization in
patients with chronic pain.[60] *This means that the division between somatogenic and psychogenic chronic pain may not be clinically productive.* Clifford
Woolf, the physician who discovered and defined the physiology of central

sensitization, has said as much in a recent review: "If activity in the forebrain circuits that drive mood and anxiety can alter nociceptive neuronal responsiveness, then this is, I consider, another cause of central sensitization, this time with a central rather than a peripheral driver."[61(p1912)] Hence, central sensitization can be both somatogenic and psychogenic.

Reconciling somatogenic and psychogenic pain: tissue danger

Lorimer Moseley and David Butler from Australia have incorporated these insights into their "Explaining Pain" program:

> Explaining Pain (EP) refers to a range of educational interventions that aim to change someone's understanding of the biological processes that are thought to underpin pain as a mechanism to reduce pain itself.... The core objective of the EP approach to treatment is to shift one's conceptualization of pain from that of a marker of tissue damage or pathology, to that of a marker of the perceived need to protect body tissue.[7(p810)]

The core insight transmitted to patients by the EP program is that the pain system is not a *damage* detection system; rather, it is a *danger* detection system. While damage can be detected on physical examination and MRI scans, danger cannot. Many features of the person's situation beyond the amount of tissue damage determine how much pain he or she will feel. This attention to the importance of context in understanding pain experience takes us well beyond the classic opposition between psychogenic and somatogenic pain.[62] Indeed, it emphasizes something about the underlying biological mechanisms of pain that is ignored by "neurophilosophers" who want to fully objectify pain: Pain is fundamentally dependent on meaning.[63]

According to Moseley and Butler, "EP emphasizes that any credible evidence of danger to body tissue can increase pain and any credible evidence of safety to body tissue can decrease pain."[7(p810)] Use of EP in a wide variety of formats has been proven to improve patients' pain and disability when added to other programs that aim to increase mobility and exercise.[64] Key messages in the EP program include the following:

- The variable relationship between nociception and pain
- The potent influence of context on pain
- Upregulation in the danger detection system as pain persists
- The fact that pain is influenced by several interacting protective systems
- Above all, the adaptability and trainability of our pain biology.

Unlike CBT and acceptance and commitment therapy (ACT), EP does challenge the reigning biomedical model concerning the causation of pain. EP moves beyond the opposition of psychogenic and somatogenic pain not only in theory, but also in practice. At this time, it has greater effects on attitudes and beliefs than on pain intensity or interference.[65] But it offers the hope of a clinically effective treatment that shifts patients' conception of pain from damage detection to danger detection.

From psychogenic pain to sociogenic pain

Utilitarian philosophers and statesmen, like Jeremy Bentham, did not distinguish pain from suffering more generally. These aversive states were targeted equally by utilitarian social policies. Poverty was just as important as back pain and other illnesses. Contemporary social scientists, like the economists Case and Deaton with their "deaths of despair" theory of the opioid epidemic, also address pain and suffering together. As economists, they are focused on economic harms like unemployment, but they recognize the special place that pain plays in our modern narrative about suffering:

> Pain has a special place in our narrative. Social and community distress, the labor market, politics, and corporate interests all collide around pain, and pain is one of the channels through which each of them affects deaths of despair. The increase in pain among less educated Americans can be traced back to the slow disintegration of their social and economic lives, and that the pain is, in turn, one of the links through which disintegration leads to suicide and addiction. The story of a death of despair often passes through pain.[66(p223)]

As the prospects for advancement through hard work have dimmed for rural White Americans without a college degree, pain problems have grown. Now middle-aged Americans report more pain than the elderly. Recent analyses show that the gap in pain between the more and less educated has widened in each successive birth cohort after 1950.[67] This pain increase is not due to changes in jobs or levels of obesity, but appears tied to the ongoing deterioration of working-class life in the United States over the past 70 years.

In the medical literature on chronic pain, we are accustomed to seeing studies of social harms like unemployment that are *caused by* chronic pain. The association of chronic low back pain with unemployment has been well known since the 19th century, when there was an epidemic of "railway spine" among railroad workers. Contemporary studies continue to document a strong relation between low back pain prevalence and unemployment rates.[68] The assumption is that back pain is causing unemployment, but this may not be the whole story. As Atul Gawande commented about Case and Deaton's analyses: "What Case and Deaton have found is that the places with a smaller fraction of the working-age population in jobs are places with higher rates of deaths of despair—and that this holds true even when you look at rates of suicide, drug overdoses, and alcohol-related liver disease separately. They all go up where joblessness does."[69(p225)] Pain and suffering go together in society. We may be able to focus on pain as a uniquely medical source of suffering within our medical institutions, but outside of these institutions, this focus is too narrow. *Separating pain from the rest of human suffering distorts human pain and human experience generally. This medicalization of pain encourages the overuse of opioids to treat human suffering.*

Since Descartes, physicians have gravitated toward physical explanations for pain problems. To explain increases in pain prevalence, we look to factors like the aging of the population or the rates of physically demanding work. But these have not provided explanations for the surge in deaths of despair among middle-aged White Americans. Increases in chronic pain do appear to be tied to changes in the labor market, but not to a shift from less physically demanding to more physically demanding work. "Low earnings are associated with more pain, and it is entirely possible that the pain comes not from what happens at work but from the loss of status and meaning as a worker, or from the loss of the social structure that was supported by a well-paying job in a union town."[66(p230)]

For example, a 2019 study has shown that automobile assembly plant closures are associated with subsequent opioid overdose mortality in that county. Counties with closures had an 85% increase in opioid mortality. Here, the *loss* of physically demanding work increases opioid mortality, not *doing* physically demanding work. These mortality increases were concentrated in working-age non-Hispanic White men.[70] A 2020 study showed that evictions also predict opioid mortality rates within a county.[71]

Someone might object that these studies only show that the social dislocations of unemployment or eviction cause drug abuse, not that they cause pain, but the population predictors of opioid misuse are also predictors of chronic pain. In the 2017 and 2018 National Survey on Drug Use and Health, these predictors included self-reported health and serious psychological distress.[72] Social dislocations are reflected in increased physical pain, which justifies opioid use. As patients grow older, physical pain relief becomes the most important reason offered for misuse of prescription opioids, with 85% of opioid misuse episodes involving pain relief as a motive.[73] Many predictors of chronic pain and opioid misuse are both biological and behavioral and can be shown to be driven by stress. These include obesity (which drives opioid prescriptions for back and joint disorders),[74] tobacco smoking (associated with pain intensity, physical functioning, opioid use and misuse),[75] and exercise (negatively associated with both joint pain and opioid use and misuse).[76,77]

Unhappiness and pain in America

Americans report greater pain than citizens of other countries, and for most subgroups of Americans happiness levels are trending downward. These are the broad conclusions of a recent book by Carol Graham, *Unhappiness for All? Unequal Hopes and Lives in Pursuit of the American Dream*.[78] She argues, based on recent Gallup World Poll and Gallup Healthways Surveys, that mental well-being has become more unequal in the United States. Specifically, she argues that America is suffering from a lack of hope, with those at the bottom of the social hierarchy becoming less hopeful about their lives and their children's lives. Notably, White Americans are now less optimistic than Black Americans. Especially those with less education have lost confidence in their chances for upward social mobility.[79] Poor Americans have more stress, more pain, and lower life satisfaction. While 20% of international samples report high pain over the past 4 weeks, 34% of Americans report high pain. We believe these trends concerning increasing pain and decreasing hope are linked, *but that this link is obscured by contemporary pain epidemiology.* We are looking for the causes of chronic pain inside the body and ignoring causes of pain outside the body.

Summary: what is wrong with the BPS model of pain?

We have spent this chapter reviewing our public health and clinical models of chronic pain because it provides us with the best overview of pain's role in our society. This includes not only the prevalence of pain but also its causes and consequences. Epidemiology provides the large-scale picture of how we conceptualize pain and its relation to other events and phenomena in our natural and cultural world. During this review, we have provided critiques of the dominant BPS model of pain, summarized in Table 5.1. We will explore them more fully in later chapters.

Table 5.1 Flaws of the BPS model

Pain issue	BPS model flaw
Causation	Does not treat biological, psychological, and social causes of chronic pain equally. Biological causes are allowed to be primary, but psychological and social causes are only allowed as modifiers. No psychogenic or sociogenic pain in the BPS model.
Medicalization	Does not address the separation of pain from suffering, including the mechanical model of pain and idea of pain as passive and innocent suffering, which supports right to pain relief and use of opioid painkillers
Pain self-management	Emphasizes managing the consequences rather than the causes of pain, in order to reduce suffering and disability rather than pain itself
Basic science	Informs multidisciplinary clinical care models for chronic pain, but not basic science models concerning etiology of pain experience. Relationship between central sensitization and psychological processes is under-investigated.
Painkillers	Accepts the pain specificity of opioid medications without addressing their psychological and social effects

Conclusion: the moral privilege of localized suffering

Both our clinical and epidemiological perspectives on pain favor causes for pain found within the body. As suggested by the research we reviewed, causal chains for chronic pain are often complicated and cyclic, crossing from inside the body to outside and back again. Toward the end of his career, pain psychologist Bill Fordyce began to call chronic pain "transdermal" in recognition of this fact. Current clinicians and researchers have given scientific priority to causes inside the body (like joint degeneration) over causes outside the body (like unemployment rates) and therefore have given higher priority to medical responses to chronic pain (like opioids) than social responses (like job training). We are willing to consider psychological and social factors as modifiers of pain biology, but not as independent pain causes.

Even more importantly, we have given *moral* priority to causes for pain and for pain experiences that can be localized in a body part. These are the pains that are more easily linked with disease or injury, and these are the pains that we see as "innocent suffering" that need medical intervention. This priority for biological causes and treatments enabled our current opioid epidemic. They have sanctioned opioid consumption for localized pain that would otherwise have been stigmatized and marginalized if taken for more diffuse suffering. In their song about heroin use, *Comfortably Numb*, the rock band Pink Floyd anticipated this localized pain justification for opioid use:

> Come on now
> I hear you're feeling down
> Well I can ease your pain
> Get you on your feet again
> Relax
> I'll need some information first
> Just the basic facts
> Can you show me where it hurts?

References

1. Merriam-Webster Dictionary. Biopsychosocial definition. 2021. https://www. merriam-webster.com/medical/biopsychosocial

2. Institute of Medicine. *Relieving Pain in America: A Blue Print for Transforming Prevention, Care, Education and Research*. National Academy of Sciences; 2011.

3. Gatchel RJ PY, Peters ML, Fuchs PN, Turk DC. The biopsychosocial approach to chronic pain: scientific advances and future directions. *Psychol Bull.* 2007;133:581–624.

4. Gatchel RJ, McGeary DD, McGeary CA, Lippe B. Interdisciplinary chronic pain management: past, present, and future. *Am Psychol.* 2014;69:119–130.

5. Rainville P, Duncan GH, Price DD, et al. Pain affect encoded in human anterior cingulate but not somatosensory cortex. *Science.* 1997;277:968–971.

6. Rainville P, Carrier B, Hofbauer RK, et al. Dissociation of sensory and affective dimensions of pain using hypnotic modulation. *Pain.* 1999;82:159–171.

7. Moseley GL, Butler DS. Fifteen years of explaining pain: the past, present, and future. *J Pain.* 2015;16:807–813.

8. Turk DC. Cognitive-behavioral approach to the treatment of chronic pain patients. *Reg Anesth Pain Med.* 2003;28:573–579.

9. Williams ACC, Fisher E, Hearn L, Eccleston C. Psychological therapies for the management of chronic pain (excluding headache) in adults. *Cochrane Database Syst Rev.* 2020;12:CD007407.

10. Tsui P DA, Yuan DY. Conversion disorder, functional neurological symptom disorder, and chronic pain: comorbidity, assessment, and treatment. *Curr Pain Headache Rep.* 2017;21:29.

11. Fordyce WE, Roberts AH, Sternbach RA. The behavioral management of chronic pain: a response to critics. *Pain.* 1985;22:113–125.

12. Carr DB, Bradshaw YS. Time to flip the pain curriculum? *Anesthesiology.* 2014;120:12–14.

13. Russo MM, Sundaramurthi T. An overview of cancer pain: Epidemiology and pathophysiology. *Semin Oncol Nurs.* 2019;35:223–228.

14. Golob AL, Wipf JE. Low back pain. *Med Clin North Am.* 2014;98:405–428.

15. McGuirk BE, Bognuk N. Low back pain. In: Ballantyne J, Fishman S, Rathmell JP, eds. *Bonica's Management of Pain*, 4th ed. Wolter Kluwers Health; 2009.

16. Deyo RA, Mirza SK. Clinical practice: herniated lumbar intervertebral disk. *N Engl J Med.* 2016;374:1763–1772.

17. Karran EL, Grant AR, Moseley GL. Low back pain and the social determinants of health: a systematic review and narrative synthesis. *Pain.* 2020;161:2476–2493.

18. Gureje O, Von Korff M, Simon GE, Gater R. Persistent pain and well-being: a World Health Organization study in primary care. *JAMA.* 1998;280:147–151.

19. Arnow BA, Hunkeler EM, Blasey CM, et al. Comorbid depression, chronic pain, and disability in primary care. *Psychosom Med.* 2006;68:262–268.

20. Katon W, Egan K, Miller D. Chronic pain: lifetime psychiatric diagnoses and family history. *Am J Psychiatry.* 1985;142:1156–1160.

21. Shaw WS, Means-Christensen AJ, Slater MA, et al. Psychiatric disorders and risk of transition to chronicity in men with first onset low back pain. *Pain Med.* 2010;11:1391–1400.

22. Hruschak V, Cochran G. Psychosocial predictors in the transition from acute to chronic pain: a systematic review. *Psychol Health Med.* 2018;23:1151–1167.

23. Wager TD, Atlas LY, Lindquist MA, et al. An fMRI-based neurologic signature of physical pain. *N Engl J Med.* 2013;368:1388–1397.

24. Engel GL. Psychogenic pain and pain-prone patient. *Am J Med.* 1959;26:899–918.

25. American Psychiatric Association. *Diagnostic and Statistical Manual of Mental Disorders.* 2nd ed. American Psychiatric Association; 1968.

26. American Psychiatric Association. *Diagnostic and Statistical Manual of Mental Disorders.* 3rd ed. American Psychiatric Association; 1980.

27. American Psychiatric Association. *Diagnostic and Statistical Manual of Mental Disorders.* 3rd ed., rev. American Psychiatric Association; 1987.

28. American Psychiatric Association. *Diagnostic and Statistical Manual of Mental Disorders.* 4th ed. American Psychiatric Association; 1994.

29. Creed F, Gureje O. Emerging themes in the revision of the classification of somatoform disorders. *Int Rev Psychiatry.* 2012;24:556–567.

30. American Psychiatric Association. *Diagnostic and Statistical Manual of Mental Disorders.* 5th ed. American Psychiatric Association; 2013.

31. Frances A, Chapman S. DSM-5 somatic symptom disorder mislabels medical illness as mental disorder. *Aust N Z J Psychiatry.* 2013;47:483–484.

32. Frances A. The new somatic symptom disorder in DSM-5 risks mislabeling many people as mentally ill. *BMJ.* 2013;346:f1580.

33. Hauser W, Wolfe F. The somatic symptom disorder in DSM 5 risks mislabelling people with major medical diseases as mentally ill. *J Psychosom Res.* 2013;75:586–587.

34. Sullivan MD. DSM-IV pain disorder: a case against the diagnosis. *Int Rev Psychiatry.* 2000;12:91–98.

35. Norris FH. Epidemiology of trauma: frequency and impact of different potentially traumatic events on different demographic groups. *J Consult Clin Psychol.* 1992;60:409–418.

36. Resnick HS, Kilpatrick DG, Dansky BS, et al. Prevalence of civilian trauma and posttraumatic stress disorder in a representative national sample of women. *J Consult Clin Psychol.* 1993;61:984–991.

37. Kessler RC, Sonnega A, Bromet E, et al. Posttraumatic stress disorder in the National Comorbidity Survey. *Arch Gen Psychiatry.* 1995;52:1048–1060.

38. Anda RF, Felitti VJ, Bremner JD, et al. The enduring effects of abuse and related adverse experiences in childhood: a convergence of evidence from neurobiology and epidemiology. *Eur Arch Psychiatry Clin Neurosci.* 2006;256:174–186.

39. Anda RF, Brown DW, Felitti VJ, et al. Adverse childhood experiences and prescription drug use in a cohort study of adult HMO patients. *BMC Public Health.* 2008;8:198.

40. Asmundson GJ, Coons MJ, Taylor S, Katz J. PTSD and the experience of pain: research and clinical implications of shared vulnerability and mutual maintenance models. *Can J Psychiatry.* 2002;47:930–937.

41. Otis JD, Keane TM, Kerns RD. An examination of the relationship between chronic pain and post-traumatic stress disorder. *J Rehabil Res Dev.* 2003;40:397–405.

42. Andreski P, Chilcoat H, Breslau N. Post-traumatic stress disorder and somatization symptoms: a prospective study. *Psychiatry Res.* 1998;79:131–138.

43. Norman SB, Stein MB, Dimsdale JE, Hoyt DB. Pain in the aftermath of trauma is a risk factor for post-traumatic stress disorder. *Psychol Med.* 2008;38:533–542.

44. Liedl A, O'Donnell M, Creamer M, et al. Support for the mutual maintenance of pain and post-traumatic stress disorder symptoms. *Psychol Med.* 2010;40:1215–1223.

45. Sullivan MJ, Thibault P, Simmonds MJ, et al. Pain, perceived injustice and the persistence of post-traumatic stress symptoms during the course of rehabilitation for whiplash injuries. *Pain.* 2009;145:325–331.

46. Seal KH, Shi Y, Cohen G, et al. Association of mental health disorders with prescription opioids and high-risk opioid use in US veterans of Iraq and Afghanistan. *JAMA.* 2012;307:940–947.

47. Langford DJ, Theodore BR, Balsiger D, et al. Number and type of post-traumatic stress disorder symptom domains are associated with patient-reported outcomes in patients with chronic pain. *J Pain.* 2018;19:506–514.

48. Hashmi JA, Baliki MN, Huang L, et al. Shape shifting pain: chronification of back pain shifts brain representation from nociceptive to emotional circuits. *Brain.* 2013;136:2751–2768.

49. Wise EA, Beck JG. Work-related trauma, PTSD, and workers compensation legislation: implications for practice and policy. *Psychol Trauma.* 2015;7:500–506.

50. Eisenberger NI, Lieberman MD, Williams KD. Does rejection hurt? An fMRI study of social exclusion. *Science.* 2003;302:290–292.

51. Eisenberger NI. The pain of social disconnection: examining the shared neural underpinnings of physical and social pain. *Nat Rev Neurosci.* 2012;13:421–434.

52. Eisenberger NI, Master SL, Inagaki TK, et al. Attachment figures activate a safety signal-related neural region and reduce pain experience. *Proc Natl Acad Sci U S A.* 2011;108:11721–11726.

53. Ciechanowski PS, Walker EA, Katon WJ, Russo JE. Attachment theory: a model for health care utilization and somatization. *Psychosom Med.* 2002;64:660–667.

54. Eisenberger NI, Jarcho JM, Lieberman MD, Naliboff BD. An experimental study of shared sensitivity to physical pain and social rejection. *Pain.* 2006;126:132–138.

55. Panksepp J, Herman B, Conner R, et al. The biology of social attachments: opiates alleviate separation distress. *Biol Psychiatry.* 1978;13:607–618.

56. Dewall CN, Macdonald G, Webster GD, et al. Acetaminophen reduces social pain: behavioral and neural evidence. *Psychol Sci.* 2010;21:931–937.

57. Woolf CJ. Central sensitization: implications for the diagnosis and treatment of pain. *Pain.* 2011;152:S2–S15.

58. Aoyagi K, He J, Nicol AL, et al. A subgroup of chronic low back pain patients with central sensitization. *Clin J Pain.* 2019;35:869–879.

59. Owens MA, Bulls HW, Trost Z, et al. An examination of pain catastrophizing and endogenous pain modulatory processes in adults with chronic low back pain. *Pain Med.* 2016;17:1452–1464.

60. McKernan LC, Johnson BN, Crofford LJ, et al. Posttraumatic stress symptoms mediate the effects of trauma exposure on clinical indicators of central sensitization in patients with chronic pain. *Clin J Pain.* 2019;35:385–393.

61. Woolf CJ. What to call the amplification of nociceptive signals in the central nervous system that contribute to widespread pain? *Pain* 2014;155:1911–1912.

62. Moseley GL, Arntz A. The context of a noxious stimulus affects the pain it evokes. *Pain.* 2007;133:64–71.

63. Arntz A, Claassens L. The meaning of pain influences its experienced intensity. *Pain.* 2004;109:20–25.

64. Moseley GL, Nicholas MK, Hodges PW. A randomized controlled trial of intensive neurophysiology education in chronic low back pain. *Clin J Pain.* 2004;20:324–330.

65. Traeger AC, Lee H, Hübscher M, et al. Effect of intensive patient education vs placebo patient education on outcomes in patients with acute low back pain: a randomized clinical trial. *JAMA Neurol.* 2019;76:161–169.

66. Case A, Deaton A. *Deaths of Despair and the Future of Capitalism.* Princeton University Press; 2020.

67. Case A, Deaton A, Stone AA. Decoding the mystery of American pain reveals a warning for the future. *Proc Natl Acad Sci U S A.* 2020;117:24785–24789.

68. Volinn E, Lai D, McKinney S, Loeser JD. When back pain becomes disabling: a regional analysis. *Pain.* 1988;33:33–39.

69. Gawande A. Why Americans are dying from despair. *New Yorker,* March 23, 2020.

70. Venkataramani AS, Bair EF, O'Brien RL, Tsai AC. Association between automotive assembly plant closures and opioid overdose mortality in the United States: A difference-in-differences analysis. *JAMA Intern Med.* 2020;180(2):254–262.

71. Bradford AC, Bradford WD. The effect of evictions on accidental drug and alcohol mortality. *Health Serv Res.* 2020;55:9–17.

72. Montiel Ishino FA, Gilreath T, Williams F. Finding the hidden risk profiles of the United States opioid epidemic: Using a person-centered approach on a national dataset of noninstitutionalized adults reporting opioid misuse. *Int J Environ Res Public Health,* 2020;17(12):4321.

73. Schepis TS, Wastila L, Ammerman B, et al. Prescription opioid misuse motives in US older adults. *Pain Med.* 2020;21(10):2237–2243.

74. Stokes A, Lundberg DJ, Sheridan B, et al. Association of obesity with prescription opioids for painful conditions in patients seeking primary care in the US. *JAMA Netw Open.* 2020;3:e202012.

75. Khan JS, Hah JM, Mackey SC. Effects of smoking on patients with chronic pain: a propensity-weighted analysis on the Collaborative Health Outcomes Information Registry. *Pain.* 2019;160:2374–2379.

76. Thanoo N, Gilbert AL, Trainor S, et al. The relationship between polypharmacy and physical activity in those with or at risk of knee osteoarthritis. *J Am Geriatr Soc.* 2020;68(9):2015–2020.

77. Dunlop DD, Song J, Semanik PA, et al. Relation of physical activity time to incident disability in community dwelling adults with or at risk of knee arthritis: prospective cohort study. *BMJ.* 2014;348:g2472.

78. Graham C. *Happiness for All? Unequal Hopes and Lives in Pursuit of the American Dream*. Princeton University Press; 2017.

79. Blanchflower DG, Oswald AJ. Unhappiness and pain in modern America: a review essay, and further evidence, on Carol Graham's *Happiness for All? J Econ Lit*. 2019;57(2):385–402.

6
Pain medicine and
the medicalization of chronic pain

Introduction: chronic pain in pain medicine

The medicalization of pain discussed in Chapters 2 and 3 was part of a shift in Western societies toward reliance on allopathic medicine to solve both the practical and existential problems of pain. Whereas acute pain and pain at the end of life have long been considered symptoms of underlying trauma or disease, treatable by primary disease management, chronic pain has not fit into the same medical model. The proposal made at the birth of the discipline of pain medicine was that chronic pain was not merely a symptom, but also a disease in its own right, needing its own specialists and its own clinics. Once chronic pain was established as a legitimate independent clinical focus, pain specialists and pain clinics abounded. Now, half a century later, chronic pain and associated disability rates are the highest on record and several medical approaches have turned out to be more harmful than helpful, while safer non-medical approaches are often dismissed in favor of the immediacy of medical approaches. One has to ask, then: Was the movement by pain medicine to medicalize chronic pain a mistake?

Jasmine Phillips, part 1

Jasmine Phillips is a 43-year-old female who suffered an injury to her right leg when she was 22 years old when she was knocked off her bike by a truck that cut across her pathway. She had fractures in her lower leg requiring an external fixator, 2 weeks in the hospital, and 3 months of rehabilitation. At the end of her rehabilitation, she was fully mobile and able to return to her job as an elder caregiver, but still had pain and was still taking a short-acting opioid.

Pain treatment harms

Medical treatment is associated with harm as well as benefit. This is true of all medical treatments. Every medical decision is based on a risk-versus-benefit analysis, and every medical treatment should be conducted so as to minimize harm. For most medical treatments, the decision is whether improvement in condition A (pneumonia) warrants the risk of developing condition B (antibiotic intolerance). For pain treatments, however, the decision is often whether improvement in condition A (pain) warrants the risk of worsening condition A (pain). For example, opioids can cause heightened pain and functional deterioration over the long term, and surgery conducted to relieve pain may actually worsen the pain. The worsening of pain with medical and surgical treatment is particularly pertinent to chronic pain care since it can respond well to non-medical approaches and self-management, albeit more slowly than it might respond to medical treatment. Examples of pain treatment worsening pain include fibromyalgia pain worsened by opioids' central effects, headache worsened by medication overuse, and joint pain worsened by steroid overuse. But perhaps there is no better example of harm from medical treatment of pain as the harm done to people with chronic back pain.

Back pain complaints are among the most common reasons for visits to primary care in the United States.[1-4] Back pain alone ranks in the top 10 of diseases or disorders contributing to the global burden of disease.[5] In the United States, total costs of lost work days due to back pain are estimated to be $100 billion to $200 billion per year.[6,7] Since back pain represents such a large portion of chronic pain, most pain clinics treat it predominantly, offering a combination of rehabilitation, interventional approaches, and medications. Along with this pain clinic evaluation, there is often an evaluation by a surgeon of the patient with back pain.

Indeed, one of the most important steps toward making back pain a disease occurred when Mixter and Barr demonstrated in 1934 that lumbar disc herniations could be surgically corrected and thereby resolve lumbar radicular pain.[8] Thus began the modern idea of considering low back pain as a surgical condition. But recent evidence has revealed that modern surgical and medical approaches to the treatment of back pain have not lowered the prevalence or population burden of back pain. Indeed, for a significant number of patients, they have made pain worse.[9]

Overuse of opioids is part of the story, and we will discuss that aspect of harm in the next chapter. But, as described in detail by Richard Deyo and colleagues, overuse of opioids is not the only iatrogenic harm done to patients with back pain.[9] Despite recommendations against routine use, rates of spinal imaging ballooned during the 1990s.[10-12] This increase has been shown to be associated with more surgery but no better clinical outcomes. U.S. medical colleges and professional groups now recommend against imaging for nonspecific low back pain (back pain without serious underlying conditions or progressive neurological deficits). However, both patients and physicians continue to request imaging, which leads to more unnecessary and possibly harmful surgery. Imaging is popular partly because physicians and health systems make money from imaging, because physicians are afraid of missing surgical lesions, and because patients love imaging. One of the only patient outcomes reliably improved by back imaging is patient satisfaction. Patients love the validation of their pain that comes with imaging. They can show these images (often with findings that are common and benign) to employers and insurance companies as well as spouses and neighbors: "Here is the cause of my pain."

Noninvasive interventions for spine pain consist largely of steroid injections into the epidural space (the tissue that surrounds and cushions the spinal cord) or into the facet joints (small joints that buttress the spinal column). These injections can have good short-term efficacy, although long-term effects are no better than natural healing. A strong argument was made that their use could reduce the need for surgery by keeping severe pain at bay and giving time for natural healing to occur. But this claim has largely been discredited by systematic reviews concluding that spinal injections do not reduce the rate of subsequent surgery.[13,14]

Invasive stimulation therapies, such as implanted spinal cord stimulators, offer a glimmer of hope for the treatment of serious, nonroutine radicular back pain, but they are expensive and only available in wealthy countries. Paradoxically, one of the best indications for spinal cord stimulation is failed back surgery syndrome. Failed back surgery syndrome arises when spine surgery that was undertaken in an attempt to relieve pain results in worse pain.

Its prevalence has been estimated at between 10% and 40% of pain-focused surgical spine cases.[15] The reason for resorting to implanted stimulation in failed back surgery syndrome is that the condition is very hard to treat and a cause of severe disabling back pain. All surgery results in scarring, and scarring can be associated with persistent pain. So perhaps it is not surprising that surgical attempts at removing whatever was causing pain in the spine, where major nerves emerge, might end up increasing pain in cases where scarring and swelling persist, or that mechanical realignment that might relieve pain in one place induces new malalignment in another. The spine is, after all, a highly complex structure that can defy simple mechanical approaches. Patients with failed back surgery syndrome have often undergone multiple surgeries, each in an attempt to correct the damage of its predecessor, with pain that can be severe, with no possibility of relief from conservative management. The tragedy of both failed back surgery syndrome and adverse opioid outcomes is that resorting to these treatments tends to impede any attempt to manage the pain conservatively. Conservative management that avoids surgery and opioids has been shown in randomized trials to result in equal or better long-term outcomes for patients with chronic back pain, even when rigorous eligibility criteria are applied.[16,17]

Pain relief becomes a product

The harm caused by zealous surgical and opioid treatment of back pain was due in part to the fact that pain relief became a product. While pain relief had always been worth paying for, now pain clinics were offering a long list of new pain-relieving technologies and products. These included ever more minimally invasive surgeries and increasingly targeted injections, for which desperate patients were willing to pay a high price. Injections and surgeries can have compelling immediate efficacy, for which people in pain and payers will pay a high price, even when cautioned that long-term benefit is unlikely.

In this business environment favoring immediate pain relief, the pharmaceutical industry spent billions of dollars developing and promoting analgesics, including opioids. Direct-to-consumer advertising, only legal in the United States and New Zealand, promoted the idea that analgesics by themselves can turn lives around, which we now know to be an unlikely and dangerous idea. The pharmaceutical industry's promotional efforts have cannily reinforced the notion that clinicians have a duty to provide their patients with pain relief. This moral pressure on primary care clinicians to provide pain relief resulted in increased resort to the prescription pad. Indeed, a prescription for opioids is one of the few interventions for chronic pain that provided immediate pain relief for the patient and a satisfied customer for the clinician. During the 1990s, the opioid prescription became the indispensable "ticket out of the exam room" where primary care providers were trapped with angry patients demanding relief of chronic pain. In the 2020s, our primary care colleagues still describe being "trapped by the pain reduction mandate" that equates chronic pain care with reduction of pain intensity scores.

What happened to pain psychology

Pain psychology and pain psychiatry were a part of the vision for multidisciplinary chronic pain care from the beginning. Bonica provided a chapter on this topic in his groundbreaking 1953 textbook. In contemporary pain medicine, the strongest clinical support for patient self-management of chronic pain is provided by pain psychology. Given that it has always held a prominent role in the ideal of multidisciplinary pain care, we must ask why psychology did not play a larger role in resisting the takeover of multidisciplinary care by opioid therapy and interventional pain clinics.

Though it is a well-researched and evidence-based treatment for chronic pain, cognitive–behavioral therapy (CBT) did not become a widely available and widely promoted commodity. There were not enough trained psychologists, insurance reimbursement was spotty, and CBT couldn't compete with pharmaceutical marketing. The time course and nature of treatment response also differed. Behavioral treatment did not produce immediate results; it was time-consuming and was often rejected by patients convinced that something in the periphery needed to be fixed. Furthermore, behavioral treatment could be perceived as stigmatizing and was often met with "you think the pain is all in my head." As behavioral treatment shrank, multidisciplinary pain management was replaced by a commercial enterprise aimed at the simpler goal of pain relief. This encouraged the growth of single-modality pain clinics focused on medical and procedural treatments that produced immediate pain relief. In the 1990s, John Bonica's groundbreaking multidisciplinary pain management received diminishing funding and support, especially from the commercial insurance plans that dominate healthcare in the United States. Behavioral approaches suffered a significant decline as the commercial enterprise of pain relief grew. Insurance companies were more willing to fund treatments that provided immediate pain relief than treatments that promoted longer-term function and return to work.

A second reason for the limited influence of pain psychology is that it has generally positioned itself as a supplement rather than an alternative to medical care for chronic pain. Patients were happy to see a medical doctor first in order to alleviate fears that a dangerous medical condition was causing the pain and to avoid the implication that their pain was "all in their head." So pain psychology did not step in until patients had been cleared medically. Furthermore, as pain medicine's goal shifted in the 1990s from management to relief, pain psychology—as supplemental—was powerless to resist the lure of pain relief.

The safety and moral necessity of pain relief through opioid therapy had been demonstrated in palliative care. If safe and effective chronic pain relief was really possible through opioid therapy, how could the psychologists resist this? Pain psychology had no persuasive answer to the promise of pain relief made on the basis of opioid pharmacology and its success in palliative care.

The high prevalence of psychopathology, especially anxiety and depression, in patients with chronic pain was well documented before the 1986 paper from Portenoy and Foley[18] and certainly before the 1996 Joint Statement on opioid therapy for chronic pain by the American Academy of Pain Medicine and the American Pain Society.[19] But the palliative care perspective interpreted these emotions as reasonable responses to serious illness and severe pain that would resolve once pain relief was provided. This consensus began to break down once the escalating rates of opioid abuse and addiction were documented. But the initial response by psychologists to emerging problems with abuse was to claim that these resulted from the prescription of opioids to people with preexisting substance abuse.[20] Some psychologists followed Purdue Pharma in claiming that the risk for opioid abuse was in the patients, not in the opioid treatment itself. It was not until the mid-2000s that pain psychology began to push back on the idea that the problem with opioid therapy originated with the "bad apples" who were prescribed this therapy.[21]

Jasmine Phillips, part 2

A year after her injury, Jasmine began complaining of new pain in her right knee, which had previously not been painful and was not injured in her accident. She told her doctor that the knee pain was worse than the surgical pain and was becoming intolerable. After several visits to her doctor, and after trying physical therapy and several non-opioid pain medications in addition to the opioid she was already taking, her doctor agreed to send her for a magnetic resonance imaging (MRI) scan of the knee. The MRI report stated that she had degenerative changes in the knee, and her doctor told her that she probably had these changes because of the stress of injury and rehabilitation. Her dose of opioid was increased, and she was told she might eventually need a knee replacement.

The demise of multidisciplinary pain management in the United States

Typically, the multidisciplinary pain clinic would comprise at least two physicians with specialty training in pain medicine, a pain psychologist, a physical therapist, and additional providers as needed (e.g., social workers, occupational therapists). Regular meetings of all the providers to discuss cases was considered an essential component of multidisciplinary care.[22] Because behavioral approaches in pain management extended into all aspects of patients' medical treatment, including their coping and living skills, the psychologist became the central figure in the Bonica-model multidisciplinary pain clinic. Psychologists were the most logical people to coordinate care among other specialists. Multidisciplinary pain management often consisted of detoxification from controlled substances (especially opioids), together with teaching self-management skills to prepare patients for a future in which they could manage pain without resort to the clinic. This way of managing complex chronic pain has been shown in several randomized trials to be the only approach with a strong evidence base supporting both immediate- and long-term benefits for pain that does not respond to simpler approaches.[23-28] Yet the model struggles to survive, especially in the United States. Just as economic factors were driving the explosive growth in single-modality pain clinics, other economic factors contributed to the inability of multidisciplinary pain clinics to survive in the new healthcare business environment.

In the 1980s, procedural codes became the way healthcare organizations billed for their services, and since services were then reimbursed on a fee-for-service basis, practitioners were encouraged to practice independently rather than in multidisciplinary groups.[3] When managed care became popular in the late 1980s, the various services could be forced into different locations and facilities, according to their lists of contracted providers. It was thus difficult to maintain the integrity of multidisciplinary care, to ensure that behavioral services were being reimbursed at competitive rates, and to get payers and patients to be patient enough to appreciate that it took time and effort to produce enduring good effects with multidisciplinary pain management.

As opioid therapy for chronic pain grew, multidisciplinary chronic pain care shrank. In 1998, there were 210 accredited multidisciplinary pain programs in the United States. By 2005, this number had dropped to 84. By 2010, it had dropped to 58. This occurred despite solid evidence of effectiveness and cost-effectiveness for these programs.[22] The rhetoric of pain relief and its business model had stronger appeal.

The one place in the United States that the multidisciplinary model has not only survived but also has been successfully integrated into primary care is military and veteran healthcare. The business model for pain care at Department of Defense (DoD) and Veterans Administration (VA) facilities is radically different than that of U.S. fee-for-service medicine. Care is capitated with widespread availability of rehabilitative, mental health, and substance abuse care. The financial incentives that drive the use of treatments with short-term benefit, like nerve blocks and opioid prescriptions, are not present. Recognizing that opioid treatment of combat injuries had begun to spill over beyond recovery, the VA led the way with its Opioid Safety Initiative, including treatment guidelines that discourage opioid use and consultative services to support non-opioid pain care provided by primary care clinicians. The VA successfully promoted and instituted stepped pain care, which not only integrates primary care with specialty care, but also addresses the psychosocial aspects of pain as primary causative and potentially remediable factors in the development of chronic pain (Figure 6.1).[29,30] The rest of the United States has not been able to recreate this thoughtful model for chronic pain care because the care organization and financial incentives to support it do not exist.

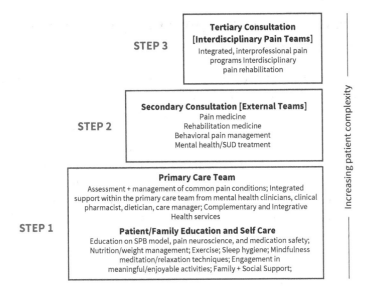

Figure 6.1. The VA Stepped-Care Model

From Mardian AS, et al. *Pain Med.* 2020;21:1168–1180, Figure 5, page 1174. License ID 1185670-1.

Jasmine Phillips, part 3

After another 18 months, Jasmine noticed pain in her left knee, and wondered if she had degenerative changes in that knee as well. When the left knee was examined, the doctor noticed that the skin over the knee had a bluish tinge and was painful to touch. The doctor wondered if she had developed complex regional pain syndrome (CRPS), a pain condition that can cross from one side to the other, occurs after injury, and makes the skin over the injury painful to touch and abnormal-looking. When the doctor examined the right knee, there were similar changes, and a diagnosis of CRPS was made. She was sent for more physical therapy, and her opioid dose was increased. She also felt unable to work and applied for disability.

An explosion of opioid prescribing in American primary care

The retreat from multidisciplinary care in the United States left primary care doctors in a difficult position. Multidisciplinary pain clinics in the Bonica model had been a resource for primary care, where their most challenging chronic pain cases could receive intensive team-based treatment that aimed to reset patients' lives. There was never enough multidisciplinary care for all who could benefit, and though many medical insurance companies were reluctant to pay for multidisciplinary care, it offered a valid treatment option for the most difficult cases. As the multidisciplinary elements in pain clinics eroded, and the team-based approach became increasingly less feasible, pain clinics adopted an increasingly interventional approach. These clinics offered advice on medications, and further specialty treatments like nerve blocks and infusions if needed, but not ongoing assistance in managing a complex chronic illness.

By the 1980s, there had been a sea change in the expectations of primary care doctors and patients concerning the management of chronic pain. Earlier, most doctors had seen pain as a symptom of disease that could usually be addressed by management of the primary disease. Pain with no obvious cause was considered "psychosomatic" or the product of "somatization" and did not receive any treatment beyond a referral to mental health professionals. Furthermore, persistent chronic pain had been seen as not suitable for opioid treatment because of opioids' limited efficacy and high risk. State laws often limited the dose and duration of opioid therapy. But as palliative care and the discipline of pain medicine began to legitimize pain as a condition in its own right, the dismissal of pain without an obvious cause as psychological became less acceptable. Clinicians were taught to believe and respect patients' reports of pain, even if no medical cause could be found—and this "respect" often took the form of a prescription for opioids.

By the 1990s, palliative care physicians had proposed the idea that if dying patients have a right to pain relief, then living patients also have this right: no one should suffer intolerable pain. Palliative and pain specialists promoted the use of a 0-to-10 pain scale that could be used as an indicator of pain severity and a need for treatment. State medical boards largely changed their policies from condemning overuse of opioids to condemning underuse. Without a viable team-based approach, primary care physicians were left exposed and alone to face patients with pain for whom they could no longer claim to have no solutions. With the stage set by this right to pain relief, the 1990s saw the pharmaceutical industry sweep in to promote its new extended-release opioid drugs in the United States as safe and effective, followed by an explosion of opioid prescribing in primary care.

Most opioid prescribing is done by primary care physicians.[31,32] This is not because primary care physicians are egregious over-prescribers, but because most chronic pain care takes place in primary care. Chronic pain is a common and enduring problem in primary care practice. One thing the opioid epidemic has taught is that no progress can be made on reducing the need to prescribe opioids and improving chronic pain management without changing the way pain is managed in primary care. Recent opioid guidelines that recommend more cautious prescribing have left primary care providers wondering what they are supposed to do now. When these providers started prescribing opioids for chronic pain in the 1990s, they seemed to be the answer to pain that could no longer be ignored or dismissed. Difficult chronic pain appeared effectively treated and patients were happy with their treatment. Years of struggling with patients who had chronic pain suddenly felt unnecessary. Opioid dose escalations were sometimes needed, but that was alright, too, because high doses were indicated according to the titrate-to-effect principle.

But then with time the darker side of the treatment emerged: the dangers of high doses, the cases of misuse and abuse, the burden to primary care clinics of desperate patients who could not keep within doses prescribed, the patients who still had pain despite high doses of opioids, and the patients who developed opioid use disorders. Opioid recommendations have now changed to favor tapering instead of upward dose titration, and primary care providers once again do not know what they are supposed to do about chronic pain and opioid problems that are actually covered by medical insurance. Opioid tapering may unmask pain, mood, and sleep problems that might be due to the original pain problem or to dependence on long-term opioid treatment or some confusing combination of both.

Jasmine Phillips, part 4

Over the next several years, Jasmine's pain escalated and spread to her hips and periodically to her shoulders and neck. Eventually she reported that she had pain all over her body, at which point her doctor diagnosed fibromyalgia. Nothing really helped, and she became socially isolated. She moved back into her parents' house after living independently with her boyfriend. Her relationship with her boyfriend ended. She consistently refused behavioral therapy, stating that her pain was not in her head. At one point, since there was nothing else to offer, her doctor suggested that a long-acting opioid might help since the dose of short-acting opioid was getting high and was not controlling the pain. At 43 years old she is taking both long- and short-acting opioids at high doses and states that the opioid is the only thing that keeps her alive. What might her life had been like if she had been discharged after her initial injury, without additional opioids? What if her doctors had not convinced her that her ongoing pain was due to something medically wrong with her leg, but instead had provided her the skills needed to cope with her continuing pain?

The multidisciplinary model of pain clinics arose out of the recognition that chronic pain is a biopsychosocial phenomenon. The model dictated a team approach that coordinated the care of its component specialists and was originally envisaged as a rehabilitation rather than a long-term care model. It provided an intensive course of multimodal treatment to address the physical, psychological, social, and medication-use aspects of chronic pain. But despite its strong evidence base, the model did not succeed broadly in the health-insurance environment of the United States, where return to work and other role functions was not valued as a healthcare outcome.[33]

Another important factor in the demise of the rehabilitation model is that it did not offer long-term pain care, which fell to primary care. Due to the continuity of primary care, it is the natural home for chronic disease management. But in the 1990s, chronic pain care in primary care was increasingly guided by palliative care and pain experts who encouraged a focus on pain intensity, patients' rights to pain relief, and the use of opioids. Since this care utilized simple assessments, the accessible prescription pad, broad medication coverage by insurance, and widely accessible pharmacies, it was much more easily implemented than multidisciplinary care. The opioid prescription seemed like a simple and easy answer for the primary care clinician who had often been trapped with angry patients asserting their right to pain relief.

Given the long-term results of these interactions and prescriptions, can the principles of multidisciplinary pain care be adapted to make it feasible in the primary care setting, where most chronic pain is treated? There is a growing recognition, since the mid-1990s, that all chronic illness (e.g., diabetes, hypertension, coronary disease, not just chronic pain) has behavioral and psychosocial contributors that can be addressed in the clinical setting. When these are not addressed, clinical care tends to be reactive instead of proactive, waiting for medical conditions to deteriorate before intervening. By 1996, chronic conditions accounted for three-quarters of healthcare costs in the United States.[34,35] Around this time, chronic disease models of care began to be developed that, similar to multidisciplinary pain care, recognized the value of team-based coordinated care. These models often involved nurses and social workers to supplement physicians, and have been widely deployed in recent decades.[36] They tend to share the essential elements of one of the first and now most-studied models—the chronic care model.[37,38] The core of this model is the active participation of patients themselves. As the authors state: "medical care for chronic illness is rarely effective in the absence of adequate self-care."[37(p1097)]

The collaborative management idea espoused by the chronic care model is based on behavioral principles: that self-management skills can be learned, that self-efficacy for these skills is important, that social environment matters, and that engaging patients in self-care improves adaptation to chronic illness. Its essential elements are (1) collaborative defining of problems (involving patient, family, and medical team), (2) targeting, goal setting, and planning, (3) creating a continuum of self-management training and support services, and (4) active, sustained follow-up. Importantly, the model does not need to be reinvented for each chronic condition. Similar models have been shown to be effective and cost-effective for many different types of chronic illnesses, including "physical illnesses" like diabetes and "mental illnesses" like depression. Like multidisciplinary pain care, it is a team-based, collaborative approach that recognizes psychosocial elements in chronic conditions and involves patients in planning and executing change. It is, by design, sustainable over the long term, following patients through the trajectory of their illnesses and their lives.

In 2021, the U.S. Agency for Healthcare Research and Quality (AHRQ) released a comparative effectiveness review on integrated pain management programs (IMPMs).[39] This review examined eight randomized controlled trials of IPMPs that were integrated into primary care settings and 49 randomized controlled trials of comprehensive pain management programs (CPMPs) that were referral-based and separate from primary care. Both the IPMPs and CPMPs showed small improvements in pain and function over the short term compared to usual care, but these faded over the intermediate to long term. CPMPs were associated with small to moderate improvements in function and pain compared to pharmacological treatment (generally nonsteroidal anti-inflammatory drugs [NSAIDs]) at multiple time points. CPMPs produced greater improvements in function, but not pain, than simple physical activity interventions. There were no differences between CPMPs and psychological therapy alone at any time. These IPMP and CPMP interventions typically include depression treatment, pain self-management training, physical reactivation, and medication management. This evidence review supports the idea that these multidisciplinary treatments are more effective than simple medication or physical activity treatments, but that the advantages are not especially large or persistent. We believe the most important conclusion of the review is that the magnitude of improvement is consistent with other treatments for chronic pain such as surgery (e.g., discectomy, vertebroplasty), steroid injections, and medications such as opioids and there is no evidence of serious or important harms. No chronic pain treatments have been shown to have large enduring effects in controlled clinical trials. There may be no "magic bullet" for chronic pain, but we have discovered that many chronic pain treatments that provide immediate relief also provide significant harm in the long term. For most patients, opioids turned out to be more a poison pill than a magic bullet.

Over the past decade, the clinical availability of accredited interdisciplinary pain rehabilitation programs similar to those tested above has continued to decline. The single exception is the VA, where accredited programs grew 10-fold, from two to 20, between 2009 and 2019. Systematic assessment of patients entering these various programs has shown significant improvements in pain, function, and quality of life.[40,41] The success of the VA model of care suggests that the organization and financing of pain care within an integrated care system can go a long way in addressing the deficits in chronic pain care that were exploited by opioid manufacturers.

The challenge of reforming chronic pain treatment in primary care still largely remains. We believe this will involve adapting the chronic care model, shown to be successful in the care of chronic illnesses like diabetes and depression, to the care of chronic pain. The hope is that by actively involving patients in their own care and in measures to maintain social, psychological, and physical wellness, the need for specialty pain care—and medications—might be substantially reduced.

Conclusion: selling a medical cure for chronic pain is iatrogenic

This chapter has examined where medical chronic pain care went wrong. It has also pointed toward the wisdom of the early pioneers in recognizing the limitations of medicine in treating pain, and in understanding pain as a biopsychosocial phenomenon that required a more personal evaluation and treatment approach. When that vision of multidisciplinary pain management was replaced by the idea that all pain needed to be relieved, the original ideals of pain medicine became corrupted. Treatments providing short-term relief with little evidence of long-term benefit (including surgery and opioids) were used increasingly, and over time began to result in harm. Underlying that harm was the claim that medicine had the cure for chronic pain when it did not. Beneath the claim that chronic pain can be cured lies a mechanical model of pain causation and a moral model of pain experience that separates pain from the remainder of human suffering as uniquely medical and uniquely innocent. We examine these models in Chapter 8.

References

1. Mantyselka P, Kumpusalo E, Ahonen R, et al. Pain as a reason to visit the doctor: a study in Finnish primary health care. *Pain.* 2001;89:175–180.
2. Breivik H, Collett B, Ventafridda V, et al. Survey of chronic pain in Europe: prevalence, impact on daily life, and treatment. *Eur J Pain.* 2006;10:287–333.
3. Tompkins DA, Hobelmann JG, Compton P. Providing chronic pain management in the "fifth vital sign" era: historical and treatment perspectives on a modern-day medical dilemma. *Drug Alcohol Depend.* 2017;173(Suppl 1):S11–S21.

4. Gaskin DJ, Richard P. The economic costs of pain in the United States. *J Pain.* 2012;13:715–724.

5. Vos T, Flaxman AD, Naghavi M, et al. Years lived with disability (YLDs) for 1160 sequelae of 289 diseases and injuries 1990-2010: a systematic analysis for the Global Burden of Disease Study 2010. *Lancet.* 2012;380:2163–2196.

6. Katz JN. Lumbar disc disorders and low-back pain: socioeconomic factors and consequences. *J Bone Joint Surg Am.* 2006;88(Suppl 2):21–24.

7. Rubin DI. Epidemiology and risk factors for spine pain. *Neurol Clin.* 2007;25:353–371.

8. Mixter WJ, Barr JS. Rupture of the intervertebral disc with involvement of the spinal canal. *N Engl J Med.* 1934;211:210–215.

9. Deyo RA, Mirza SK, Turner JA, Martin BI. Overtreating chronic back pain: time to back off? *J Am Board Fam Med.* 2009;22:62–68.

10. Swedlow A, Johnson G, Smithline N, Milstein A. Increased costs and rates of use in the California workers' compensation system as a result of self-referral by physicians. *N Engl J Med.* 1992;327:1502–1506.

11. Rao JK, Kroenke K, Mihaliak KA, et al. Can guidelines impact the ordering of magnetic resonance imaging studies by primary care providers for low back pain? *Am J Manag Care.* 2002;8:27–35.

12. Schroth WS, Schectman JM, Elinsky EG, Panagides JC. Utilization of medical services for the treatment of acute low back pain: conformance with clinical guidelines. *J Gen Intern Med.* 1992;7:486–491.

13. Airaksinen O, Brox JI, Cedraschi C, et al. European guidelines for the management of chronic nonspecific low back pain. *Eur Spine J.* 2006;15(Suppl 2):S192–S300.

14. Armon C, Argoff CE, Samuels J, Backonja MM. Assessment: use of epidural steroid injections to treat radicular lumbosacral pain: report of the Therapeutics and Technology Assessment Subcommittee of the American Academy of Neurology. *Neurology.* 2007;68:723–729.

15. Inoue S, Kamiya M, Nishihara M, et al. Prevalence, characteristics, and burden of failed back surgery syndrome: the influence of various residual symptoms on patient satisfaction and quality of life as assessed by a nationwide internet survey in Japan. *J Pain Res.* 2017;10:811–823.

16. Weinstein JN, Tosteson TD, Lurie JD, et al. Surgical vs. nonoperative treatment for lumbar disk herniation: the Spine Patient Outcomes Research Trial (SPORT): a randomized trial. *JAMA.* 2006;296:2441–2450.

17. Krebs EE, Gravely A, Nugent S, et al. Effect of opioid vs. nonopioid medications on pain-related function in patients with chronic back pain or hip

or knee osteoarthritis pain: The SPACE randomized clinical trial. *JAMA.* 2018;319:872–882.

18. Portenoy RK, Foley KM. Chronic use of opioid analgesics in non-malignant pain: report of 38 cases. *Pain.* 1986;25:171–186.

19. Dersh J, Polatin PB, Gatchell RJ. Chronic pain and psychopathology: research finding and theoretical considerations. *Psychom Med.* 2002;64:773–786.

20. Passik S, Kirsh K. The need to identify predictors of aberrant drug-related behavior and addiction in patients being treated with opioids for pain. *Pain Med.* 2003;4:186–189.

21. Turk DC, Swanson KS, Gatchel RJ. Predicting opioid misuse by chronic pain patients: a systematic review and literature synthesis. *Clin J Pain/* 2008;24:497–508.

22. Gatchel RJ, McGeary DD, McGeary CA, Lippe B. Interdisciplinary chronic pain management: past, present, and future. *Am Psychol.* 2014;69:119–130.

23. Flor H, Fydrich T, Turk DC. Efficacy of multidisciplinary pain treatment centers: a meta-analytic review. *Pain.* 1992;49:221–230.

24. Kamper SJ, Apeldoorn AT, Chiarotto A, et al. Multidisciplinary biopsychosocial rehabilitation for chronic low back pain: Cochrane systematic review and meta-analysis. *BMJ.* 2015;350:h444.

25. Roberts AH, Sternbach RA, Polich J. Behavioral management of chronic pain and excess disability: long-term follow-up of an outpatient program. *Clin J Pain.* 1993;9:41–48.

26. Patrick LE, Altmaier EM, Found EM. Long-term outcomes in multidisciplinary treatment of chronic low back pain: results of a 13-year follow-up. *Spine.* 2004;29:850–855.

27. Linssen AC, Spinhoven P. Multimodal treatment programmes for chronic pain: a quantitative analysis of existing research data. *J Psychosom Res.* 1992;36:275–286.

28. Murphy JL, Schatman ME. Interdisciplinary chronic pain management: perspectives on history, current status, and future viability. In: Ballantyne JC, Fishman SM, Rathmell JR, eds. *Bonica's Management of Pain.* Wolters Kluwer; 2018:1709–1716.

29. Becker WC, Edmond SN, Cervone DJ, et al. Evaluation of an integrated, multidisciplinary program to address unsafe use of opioids prescribed for pain. *Pain Med.* 2018;19:1419–1424.

30. Edmond SN, Moore BA, Dorflinger LM, et al. Project STEP: Implementing the Veterans Health Administration's stepped care model of pain management. *Pain Med.* 2018;19:S30–S37.

31. Desveaux L, Saragosa M, Kithulegoda N, Ivers NM. Family physician percep-
    tions of their role in managing the opioid crisis. *Ann Fam Med.* 2019;17:345–351.
32. Ringwalt C, Gugelmann H, Garrettson M, et al. Differential prescribing of
    opioid analgesics according to physician specialty for Medicaid patients with
    chronic noncancer pain diagnoses. *Pain Res Manag.* 2014;19:179–185.
33. Schatman ME. The role of the health insurance industry in perpetuating subop-
    timal pain management. *Pain Med.* 2011;12:415–426.
34. Hoffman C, Rice D, Sung HY. Persons with chronic conditions: their prevalence
    and costs. *JAMA.* 1996;276:1473–1479.
35. World Health Organization. *Preventing Chronic Diseases: A Vital Investment.*
    World Health Organization; 2005.
36. Grover A, Joshi A. An overview of chronic disease models: a systematic litera-
    ture review. *Glob J Health Sci.* 2014;7:210–227.
37. Von Korff M, Gruman J, Schaefer J, et al. Collaborative management of chronic
    illness. *Ann Intern Med.* 1997;127:1097–1102.
38. Wagner EH, Austin BT, Von Korff M. Organizing care for patients with chronic
    illness. *Milbank Q.* 1996;74(4):511–544.
39. Agency for Healthcare Research and Quality. *Comparative Effectiveness Review,
    Number 251, Integrated Pain Management Programs.* U.S. Government Printing
    Office; 2021. https://effectivehealthcare.ahrq.gov/sites/default/files/pdf/cer-
    251-integrated-pain-management.pdf
40. Bair MJ, Ang D, Wu J, et al. Evaluation of Stepped Care for Chronic Pain
    (ESCAPE) in veterans of the Iraq and Afghanistan conflicts: a randomized clin-
    ical trial. *JAMA Intern Med.* 2015;175:682–689.
41. Murphy JL, Palyo SA, Schmidt ZS, et al. The resurrection of interdisciplinary
    pain rehabilitation: outcomes across a Veterans Affairs collaborative. *Pain Med.*
    2021;22:430–443.

7
Selling opioids as targeted painkillers

Introduction: understanding pain requires understanding opioids

While we have discussed the adaptation of opioid therapy from palliative care to chronic pain care in previous chapters, our focus has been on our understanding of pain as a problem in society, the selling of the product of pain relief, and the origins of the right to pain relief. But it is not possible to fully understand the problem of pain without understanding the functions of the brain's endogenous opioid system. Until this system was discovered in 1973 by Candace Pert and Solomon Snyder, the pain-relieving properties of poppy-derived opioids were thought to be a happy accident or a gift from God. But once Pert and Snyder discovered specific opioid receptors in the brain, and others discovered the endogenous opioids (e.g., endorphins, enkephalins, dynorphins) that activated these receptors, it became clear that opioids were part of the normal functioning of the human brain. These endogenous opioids do indeed provide pain relief, but they do much more than this. They are one of the main stress modulators in the brain. They help integrate the brain's punishment and reward systems. And they support uniquely human social and emotional function. This means that it is a serious error to understand opioids, endogenous and exogenous, as only painkillers.

Phoebe Nash, part 1

Phoebe Nash would be the first to say that her whole identity had become tied up in her work. She was the first in her family to go to college, and she had loved the college experience. Most of her friends were women, and

> they would meet to go over their work and discuss what they were reading about and learning. They would often stay up discussing well into the night. Occasionally they would eat together, but mostly their friendships were centered on their studies. After she graduated, Phoebe decided to pursue a PhD, so she stayed on at college and did paid teaching to support herself while she prepared her dissertation. By the time she was 35, she had become a professor of English literature, still lived on campus, and continued to focus her whole life on her work. She was by nature fiercely independent, but she had a few good friends, and when she traveled, she usually did so with a friend.

In modern medicine, we have separated pain as a mechanically produced medical problem from the rest of human suffering. Medical professionals have embraced opioids as an essential tool in the effort to control this pain. This has been very successful in limited medical contexts such as acute postoperative and posttraumatic pain or end-of-life pain. But use in chronic pain care, which is not limited in time and/or limited to patients in medical institutions, has shown that understanding opioids as painkillers is dangerously inadequate. All the diverse and important functions of endogenous opioids are affected when the human brain is exposed to continuous exogenous opioid therapy for months, years, or decades.

The early history of opioids in Europe and America

Opioids played little role in the transformation of pain from a religious problem into a social problem that occurred in Europe between 1500 and 1800. This is because prescribed medications, or drugs of any kind, did not play a significant role in addressing the social problem of pain in Europe during the 16th, 17th, and 18th centuries.

Paracelsus (1494–1541) was a Swiss physician and alchemist, as well as a lay theologian and philosopher, who participated in the German Renaissance. He introduced mercury as a treatment for syphilis. He is also reported to be the first to bring laudanum (tincture of opium in ethanol) back to Europe from Arabia in 1527. But the use of opium in medical practice remained unusual for at least a century after this.

In 1680, Thomas Sydenham (Figure 7.1), known as the "English Hippocrates," recommended laudanum for pain, sleeplessness, and diarrhea: "Among the remedies which it has pleased Almighty God to give to man to relieve his sufferings, none is so universal and so efficacious as opium." In the 18th century, opium was widely used for cholera, dysentery, and cough, and was also found useful for nervous disorders and insomnia. Indeed, opium was a benign alternative to the arsenics, mercuries, and other toxic treatments in use at the time, and it appeared successful in alleviating a remarkably wide range of ailments.

By the 19th century, opium was used more broadly for pain, especially for the "female complaints" of hysteria and neurasthenia. This practice was criticized because neurasthenia was thought to predispose women to opium addiction. Indeed, it is estimated that there were 150,000 to 200,000

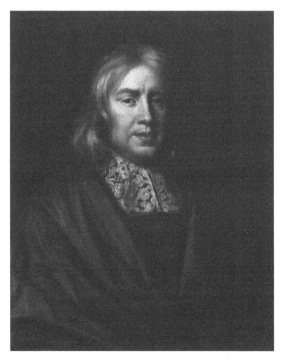

Figure 7.1. Portrait of Thomas Sydenham (1624–1689) by Mary Beale
Public domain

opiate addicts in the United States in the late 19th century, most of whom were women.[1] The modern era of opiate prescribing began when morphine was synthesized in 1803, then sold commercially in 1827. The hypodermic needle and syringe were invented in the 1850s. Morphine was used widely in the American Civil War and many soldiers returned home addicted to it. By the end of the 19th century, America was in the midst of its first opioid epidemic.

By the end of the 20th century, the social significance of opioid therapy had changed. Indeed, some of the earliest and most vocal advocates of opioid therapy for chronic pain spoke of it providing benefits, not just for individual patients, but also for the overall population. In 2004, Dr. Russell Portenoy stated, "For those who interpreted a rise in prescribing as a necessary step in the broader effort to address the problem of unrelieved pain, the growth in opioid prescribing was a gratifying trend."[2(p739)] Wider opioid prescribing was welcomed as a strategy to lower the overall level of pain and suffering in society. The early advocates of opioid therapy had worked in palliative care, where they had become convinced that allowing patients to *die* in overwhelming pain was unethical and abhorrent. They came to believe that allowing patients with chronic pain to *live* in overwhelming pain was also unethical and abhorrent. Through liberalizing access to opioids, they sought to lift the burden of overwhelming pain from these patients, thereby reducing the burden of pain for society as a whole.

Phoebe Nash, part 2

Not long after her 35th birthday, Phoebe noticed double vision. Her doctor told her it was probably stress, and that she should try to incorporate exercise and stress reduction into her life. The double vision fluctuated, but it was still worrying, particularly when she also noticed weakness in her right leg, and difficulty walking. She was diagnosed with multiple sclerosis (MS) not long after the onset of difficulty walking. Sadly, despite treatment, her disease progressed very rapidly, and by the time she was 40 years old, she was wheelchair dependent. She became quite depressed, believing that she had lost her teaching career. But antidepressant medication and psychotherapy helped her see that she was still able to teach.

She told her friends and her physicians that she could cope with all the changes that the disease had wrought, as long as she could continue her teaching, reading and research, and publishing papers. She had burning pain in her legs, but she could cope with that too, as long as it did not interfere with her work. But gradually the pain worsened, and none of the medications she had been given prevented the pain from interfering with her sleep and her ability to work.

Opioids' role in pain medicine failures

Perhaps no area of pain medicine better illustrates how medical treatment can harm as well as help than the use of opioids. Opioids are, of course, an age-old treatment for pain. They can still be considered the most effective analgesic medications available, at least in the short term, despite the introduction of many newer pain-relieving medications. Yet, the harm related to their medical use is also well known. Because they are highly addictive, especially if not taken under medical control, their spread into communities can have far-reaching adverse impact. This occurs largely through the spread of addiction and its effects on people's ability to function normally as individuals, in relationships, and in society. In addition, opioids have dangerous side effects, especially respiratory depression, capable of causing death. Dangerous side effects of opioids occur during medical treatment as well as during non-medical use. We have argued throughout this book that the current U.S. opioid epidemic was not caused by opioids alone. Rather, turning to opioids for pain relief at an unprecedented level during the past few decades was a consequence of much higher expectation for obtaining relief through medical intervention.

Throughout the 20th century, not only were attitudes to pain changing, but attitudes to opioids as medical treatment were also changing, and these changes had a profound effect on their medical use. At the onset of the 20th century, opioid addiction, arising in no small part from domestic use of laudanum (opioid elixir) to treat pain, had become so widespread in the United States and Europe that it was felt necessary to restrict opioid use.[3] In the United States, the Harrison Act, introduced in 1914, for the first time made it illegal to produce, distribute, or use opioids and other addictive drugs other than by medical prescription.[4] Over a century later, we take it for granted that any opioid use other than that prescribed by a medical practitioner is illegal. But before the Harrison Act, opioids were freely available to anyone who wished to purchase them, and the choice to use opioids for the treatment of pain was up to the conscience of the individual, not up to the judgment of a physician. Alethea Hayter, in her book *Opium and the Romantic Imagination*, compares opium use in Victorian England to opioid use today:

> No one who thinks of the early nineteenth-century opium addicts in terms of what their position would be today—forced to pester reluctant doctors daily for a barely sufficient dose, or to pay large sums for illicit supplies, in danger of prosecution and of blackmail—will be able to understand the frame of mind of someone like Coleridge [poet and opium addict Samuel Taylor Coleridge], who had no obstacles between him and drug but his own conscience and the reproaches of his immediate family and closest friends; no difficulty and little expense in getting supplies, no public opprobrium, no legal danger, a divided opinion among doctors about the merits and dangers of the drug and many widely-read travel books about the opium eaters of the East to stimulate curiosity and experiment.[5(p28)]

In one stroke, the Harrison Act drug regulations passed the moral and ethical burden of the choice to use opioids to physicians. Opioid use was thereby condemned if used for any reason other than the treatment of bodily pain. But in reality, physical and emotional pain cannot be so neatly divided. Opioid use, whether licit or illicit, could be chosen for the treatment of bodily pain, but even if this is the reason that opioids are chosen, opioids do not simply target bodily pain. Opioid medications affect a wide range of survival mechanisms, and produce wide-ranging neuroadaptations over time. These changes alter people's stress responses, mood, energy, and drive, and thereby alter people's behaviors. With long-term use, these changes may not differ greatly between pain patients and people using opioids illicitly.[6,7] Although regulations try to draw a line between prescribed and nonprescribed opioid use, this line cannot separate intended from unintended opioid functions within the brain. Drug regulations had essentially created an imaginary boundary between physical and emotional pain, and in doing so, narrowed the scope of decision-making on opioid use for both the person and the clinician.

Phoebe Nash, part 3

Nobody wanted to give Phoebe opioids, but her level of distress was so extreme that the physician looking after her MS relented and started her on a low dose of oxycodone. She had convinced her physician that her life was not worth living unless she could work, and she was sure she would be able to work again if only she had some pain relief. She still maintained her independence. In fact, an unspoken fear that her disease, and maybe her pain, would eventually disable her, made her reject offers of help from both friends and family. After all, being a strong person was part of who she was.

The opioid treatment was life-changing. She felt a huge burden had lifted. She was able to sleep through the night, and wake up feeling refreshed and rested. She got back her ability to concentrate, study, and write. And she no longer feared she might not be able to get through her teaching sessions as the pain became more and more unbearable. She was so grateful to her physician for "making my life worth living again." At each visit, she told her physician how grateful she was for the pain relief.

The Harrison Act and its amendments enshrined in U.S. policy an understanding of opioids as painkillers that, if misused, could be addictive. Legitimate opioid use occurred when opioids were prescribed by doctors for pain control. Illegitimate opioid abuse occurred when people took unprescribed opioids for any reason, but especially for non-medical mood manipulation. This understanding of opioids as potentially addictive painkillers is challenged (in ways we are only still coming to understand) by the discovery in the 1970s of an endogenous (within the body) opioid system.[8,9] The endogenous opioid system consists of hormone-like mediators (endorphins and enkephalins) that act through receptors throughout the body but mostly in the brain and nervous system. Once it was understood that opioid drugs worked through people's own endogenous opioid systems, it gradually became clear that the pain-relieving and rewarding effects of opioid drugs are not distinct and separate, but are integrated and interdependent.[10]

The endogenous opioid system, as an evolved human brain system, is focused on survival.[11] The multiple functions of the endogenous opioid system, such as relief of pain, slowing of breathing, slowing of bowel movements, and rewarding of survival behaviors (including feeding, mating, and social bonding, to name just a few), are all necessary for human survival. Other non-mammalian species have rudimentary endogenous opioid systems focused on pain control, but these are primitive compared to the human system. None of these other systems are as complex or as involved in complex socialization as in humans, for whom survival depends on social networking.[12-14] These human systems not only become active during fight and flight, they are also constantly at work adapting to the environment, sensing what is injurious both physically and emotionally, and working to restore homeostasis most of the time.

There are diverse human endogenous opioid functions encompassing not only pain and reward but appetitive behaviors of many types, neuroendocrine and reproductive functions, and balancing the stress response with the need to restore and rebuild after stress relents. Different parts of our brains and nervous systems are activated for different roles, and different levels of activity. The varied endogenous opioid actions are integrated and interdependent with these.

Phoebe Nash, part 4

A year of opioid therapy went by, and the physician began to feel that despite having had trepidation, prescribing an opioid had been the right thing to do. But after another year, Phoebe began to complain that the dose that had been working well was no longer enough. The dose was still within guideline-recommended limits, so the physician increased the dose. Two further dose increases were still within the limits, but the dose was increasing and occasionally even the higher dose was not enough to last between prescriptions. Phoebe started having more depression and more pain, with difficulty sleeping and difficulty concentrating, just as she had before she started taking opioids. In fact, both these difficulties just seemed to be getting worse and worse. Was the disease getting worse, or was the opioid just not doing the job it did before because of opioid tolerance? Would a higher opioid dose help? What worried her physician the most now was that she had stopped going into work, and whereas she had always been very well groomed, she had begun to look disheveled, and she was losing weight. After years of fierce independence, she agreed to let her mother come and look after her. Phoebe still believed that she was far better off than she would be if she was taken off opioids.

Opioid drugs (exogenous opioids), on the other hand, cannot achieve such targeting or subtlety as is characteristic of the endogenous system. Instead of fine-tuning to the overall benefit of the organism or person, exogenous opioids act throughout the whole endogenous opioid system, and are themselves incapable of adjusting to circumstance or need. Instead, exogenous opioid actions are dependent on dose and the person's adaptation to the drug. Moreover, opioid drugs commandeer the endogenous system, so that the person may have difficulty mounting beneficial endogenous effects such as pain relief, natural rewards, and, importantly, the rewarding effects of socialization. The chronic opioid user, whether such use is therapeutic or not, will tend to look to further drug use for the positive effects of pain relief and reward, rather than to the more natural alternatives such as exercise, laughter, music, meditation, touch, close relationships, and friendships, all of which stimulate the endogenous opioid system.

With chronic drug use the human opioid system adapts. Our endogenous system will attempt to adapt to the opioid drug just as it does to natural events. The most obvious expression of such neuroadaptation is drug tolerance. Drug tolerance can appear as a need for a higher dose to achieve the same effect, or if tolerance is not matched with more drug, can appear as withdrawal or drug dependence. But these relatively simple clinical manifestations belie the complexity of the underlying adaptations. As with any drug tolerance, part of the tolerance arises through desensitization at the receptor level.[15] But opioids, as drugs that have hedonic (pleasing) effects, also engender more complex adaptations that counteract their pleasing effects.[16] These adaptations function by attempting to restore physiological and emotional homeostasis (stability). But in responding to exogenous opioid drugs, the adaptive response may be of much greater magnitude and less targeted than normal adaptations.

Since the nervous system's adaptation opposes the drug's hedonic and pain-relieving effects, the withdrawal consists of not only classical physical effects such as nausea, agitation, and goose bumps, but also emotional effects such as insensitivity to pleasure and increased sensitivity to pain. The classic physical opioid withdrawal largely results from the recovery of desensitizing effects and disappears within days. The latter emotional effects may take weeks or years to recover.

Opponent effects explain a lot about opioid dependence and addiction. When a patient continues to take opioids, they induce adaptations that, as drug-opposite effects, make it hard to live without opioids. Long-term sequelae of adaptations may mean life-long dependence on opioids. Pain relief that is initially helpful often turns into pain relief that can only be maintained through dose escalation. Dose tapering may be too distressing to be tolerated, as wide-ranging opponent effects can take months or years to recover.

Phoebe Nash, part 5

When her mother went with Phoebe to the first medical appointment after moving in to look after her daughter, she told the physician that her daughter was just not herself, and she was very worried about her dependence on opioids. She said that her daughter had gone from being self-sufficient to dependent rapidly, and she was worried it was the opioid use that was the problem, not so much the disease. The disease symptoms did not seem to have progressed, but she no longer had any desire to work or look after herself. Moreover, at the end of each dosing period, she became desperate for the next dose, often took early doses, and often ran out of medication early. By now the opioid dose was higher than guidelines recommended, and the physician began to worry that the doses were harming her.

The physician tried to have a conversation about tapering, but the conversation produced so much distress that the physician backed off, and in fact backed off several more times before sending Phoebe to a pain clinic. It had been tempting to start opioids, and for a while it seemed to have been the right decision. But Phoebe, like so many other opioid-treated patients with chronic pain, ultimately became tolerant and dependent, was no longer getting much benefit, and was likely being changed as a person by her opioid use, since opioids numb everything, not just pain. She was now in a tough spot because it is not easy to get someone off established opioid therapy.

Opioid policy forgets the endogenous opioid system

Since the discovery of an endogenous opioid system in the 1970s vastly expanded our knowledge of pain and addiction interdependence, how was it possible that by the early 1990s the medical community was convinced that opioids given for pain would be minimally addictive?[17] In part, this was due to the success of the palliative care movement in establishing opioids as safe and effective. The pharmaceutical industry then disseminated this message into not just medical education, but also policy, regulation, and law. The industry's fundamental tactic was to convince people to abandon the fear that chronic opioid use was ineffective and unsafe. This was buttressed by the idea that withholding opioids was bad medicine, even unethical. This tactic succeeded beyond anyone's wildest dream, and opioid prescribing, at least in the United States, increased fourfold in the ensuing years.[18] It was not until two decades later that we recognized that the increase in prescribing for pain had triggered an epidemic of opioid abuse and deaths.

What most worried people about opioids was the increase in abuse admissions and opioid-related deaths. But what our knowledge of endogenous opioid actions should have triggered is much greater concern about the underlying social consequences of widespread opioid use. These social consequences are reflected not only in abuse admissions or deaths. Opioid social and emotional impairments affect a far greater number of individuals than those who become addicted or who overdose. Opioids not only relieve pain but also deactivate people. Economist Alan Krueger has attributed a large percentage of workforce nonparticipation (disability plus unemployment) among working-age Americans to opioid use. Opioid dependence will occur with long-term continuous opioid use, leaving users socially detached and isolated. They will lose their libido, energy, and drive, and will tend to choose passivity rather than action (such as exercise and engagement in work, career, family, and home building). Widespread opioid pain treatment has had a corrosive effect on U.S. society,[19] not only because of addiction, but also because of damage to important endogenous mechanisms that sustain normal human life and socialization.

Adverse selection: result of the failed effort to target opioid therapy at physical pain

Opioid treatment guidelines have urged prescribers to carefully screen potential opioid recipients for substance use and mental health disorders, ostensibly to avoid fostering addiction in these vulnerable patients. The implicit purpose of this risk stratification procedure was to aim opioid therapy at physical pain and away from social and emotional pain. This effort failed dramatically; in fact, the opposite has occurred. Many studies have demonstrated that patients with substance use and mental health disorders are more likely to prescribed opioids, at higher doses, over longer periods of time, and often with concurrent sedatives.[20] We have used the term "adverse selection" to describe how opioids were distributed when they were widely prescribed. Adverse selection describes the paradoxical fact that the individuals at highest risk for bad outcomes (due to concurrent substance use and mental health disorders) are those who tend to be prescribed the highest-risk opioid regimens. It may seem obvious that individuals with these risk factors would be more likely to experience bad opioid outcomes. But this does not explain why these individuals would be prescribed the riskiest high-dose opioid regimens. What the medical community did not understand is that substance use and mental health disorders increase both the desire for opioids and the risk of developing chronic pain. The patients with substance use and mental health disorders seek out opioid therapy for chronic pain somewhat more avidly than those without these disorders. But they are much more likely to stay on opioids long term and to escalate doses over time.[21]

Doctors and their patients have tended to see physical pain as imposed and mechanical—that is, as passive suffering originating outside the person. But that ignores the fact that what we call "pain" is a personal perception that only arises once the pain stimulus (or nociceptive input) has been processed by the brain and spinal cord.[22,23] That is why reported pain shows enormous variation, correlated much more closely with the person than with the stimulus. In other words, something about the person determines the pain experience, regardless of the nociceptive input.

What neuroscientists have been able tell us is that the person, or particularly the person's homeostatic stress response, is profoundly changed by past events. Traumatic events, particularly repeat or severe traumatic events, engender permanent alterations in stress responses, or allostasis.[24,25] Allostasis is now believed to underlie many chronic diseases, including chronic pain. Both pain and addictive disorders are characterized by impaired capacity for pleasure, compulsive drug-seeking, and high stress. One important component of such changed stress responses is a change in opioid responsivity. The endogenous opioid system becomes over-stimulated and develops what some neuroscientists have termed heightened "opioid tone," a state equivalent to being on exogenous opioids and being constantly on the verge of withdrawal.[26-28] High opioid tone has been found in nociplastic pain syndromes such as fibromyalgia. High "opioid tone" paradoxically makes the person want opioids, and feel more than the usual amount of relief when opioids are taken.[29] These concepts, illustrated in Figure 7.2, help us understand why patients reporting the most severe pain and the greatest psychiatric comorbidity, tend to have the worst outcomes when they take opioids for the treatment of their chronic pain.

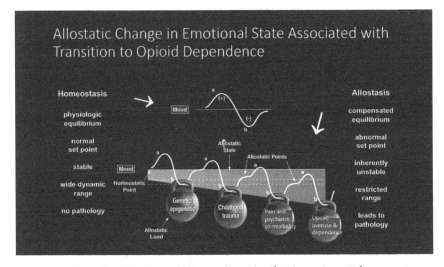

Figure 7.2. From Koob GF. Drug addiction: hyperkatifeia/negative reinforcement as a framework for medications development. *Pharmacol Rev.* 2021;73:163–201, Figure 6, page 188. License ID 1183535-1. Written permission obtained from George Koob for modification.

Conclusion: opioids are not simple painkillers

The late-20th-century embrace and overuse of opioid pain treatment in many senses resulted from the failed promise of pain medicine. It all started with drug regulation, which separated legitimate medical use (where opioids were prescribed for physical pain) from illegitimate non-medical use (where opioids were often used to counter psychological and social pain). Physicians were to limit opioid prescriptions to patients with physical pain. All industry and pain advocates had to do then was persuade physicians it was just and necessary to prescribe for physical pain, and that this pain was completely distinct from the risk of addiction. Industry's route to greater sales was persuasion of physicians, greater production and greater distribution of opioids, and activation of a profit-driven pain relief system, with the result that unprecedented amounts of prescription opioids were suddenly available for both use and abuse. It was a brilliant marketing tactic because the reliability and immediacy of opioid pain relief meant that opioids produced results when other treatments had failed or were too slow to show benefit.

Given what we know about the varied functions of the endogenous opioid system, it is not surprising that opioid therapy addressed the trauma and distress of the most vulnerable people with chronic pain. Our error was believing that opioids could be targeted to relieve physical pain specifically. This error about opioids is a special case of a more general error that separates our understanding of pain from our understanding of suffering more generally. We turn our attention to this more general error in our next chapter.

References

1. Courtwright DT. The hidden epidemic: opiate addiction and cocaine use in the South, 1860–1920. *J South Hist*. 1983;49:57–72.
2. Portenoy RK. Appropriate use of opioids for persistent non-cancer pain. *Lancet*. 2004;364:739–740.
3. Manchikanti L, Sanapati J, Benyamin RM, et al. Reframing the prevention strategies of the opioid crisis: focusing on prescription opioids, fentanyl, and heroin epidemic. *Pain Physician*. 2018;21:309–326.
4. Harrison Narcotics Tax Act https://www.druglibrary.org/schaffer/history/e1910/harrisonact.htm

5. Hayter A. *Opium and the Romantic Imagination*. Faber and Faber; 1968.

6. Gallagher RM, Koob GF, Popescu A. The pathophysiology of chronic pain and clinical interfaces with addiction. In: Ries RK, Fiellin DA, Miller SC, Saitz R, eds. *ASAM Principles of Addiction Medicine*. 5th ed. Wolters Kluwer; 2014:1435–1456.

7. Shurman J, Koob GF, Gutstein HB. Opioids, pain, the brain, and hyperkatifeia: a framework for the rational use of opioids for pain. *Pain Med*. 2010;11:1092–1098.

8. Hughes J, Smith TW, Kosterlitz HW, et al. Identification of two related pentapeptides from the brain with potent opiate agonist activity. *Nature*. 1975;258:577–580.

9. Pert CB, Snyder SH. Opiate receptor binding of agonists and antagonists affected differentially by sodium. *Mol Pharmacol*. 1974;10:868–879.

10. Cahill CM, Cook C, Pickens S. Migraine and reward system—or is it aversive? *Curr Pain Headache Rep*. 2014;18:410.

11. Ballantyne JC, Sullivan MD. Discovery of endogenous opioid systems: what it has meant for the clinician's understanding of pain and its treatment. *Pain*. 2017;158:2290–2300.

12. Panksepp J, Herman B, Conner R, et al. The biology of social attachments: opiates alleviate separation distress. *Biol Psychiatry*. 1978;13:607–618.

13. Carr DB. Endogenous opioids' primary role: harmonizing individual, kin/cohort, and societal behaviors. *Pain Med*. 2017;18:201–203.

14. Carr DB, Bradshaw YS. Time to flip the pain curriculum? *Anesthesiology*. 2014;120:12–14.

15. Williams JT, Ingram SL, Henderson G, et al. Regulation of mu-opioid receptors: desensitization, phosphorylation, internalization, and tolerance. *Pharmacol Rev*. 2013;65:223–254.

16. Koob GF. Drug addiction: hyperkatifeia/negative reinforcement as a framework for medications development. *Pharmacol Rev*. 2021;73:163–201.

17. Boudreau D, Von Korff M, Rutter CM, et al. Trends in long-term opioid therapy for chronic non-cancer pain. *Pharmacoepidemiol Drug Saf*. 2009;18:1166–1175.

18. Paulozzi LJ, Ryan GW. Opioid analgesics and rates of fatal drug poisoning in the United States. *Am J Prev Med*. 2006;31:506–511.

19. Case A, Deaton A. Rising morbidity and mortality in midlife among white non-Hispanic Americans in the 21st century. *Proc Natl Acad Sci U S A*. 2015;112:15078–15083.

20. Sullivan MD, Edlund MJ, Zhang L, et al. Association between mental health disorders, problem drug use, and regular prescription opioid use. *Arch Intern Med*. 2006;166:2087–2093.

21. Sullivan MD. Depression effects on long-term prescription opioid use, abuse, and addiction. *Clin J Pain*. 2018;34:878–884.

22. Baliki MN, Petre B, Torbey S, et al. Corticostriatal functional connectivity predicts transition to chronic back pain. *Nat Neurosci*. 2012;15:1117–1119.

23. Apkarian AV, Baliki MN, Geha PY. Towards a theory of chronic pain. *Prog Neurobiol*. 2009;87:81–97.

24. Sterling P, Eyer J. Allostasis: a new paradigm to explain arousal pathology. In: Fisher S, Reason J, eds. *Handbook of Life Stress, Cognition and Health*. John Wiley; 1988:629–649.

25. Peters A, McEwen BS. Introduction for the allostatic load special issue. *Physiol Behav*. 2012;106:1–4.

26. White JM. Pleasure into pain: the consequences of long-term opioid use. *Addict Behav*. 2004;29:1311–1324.

27. Chaijale NN, Curtis AL, Wood SK, et al. Social stress engages opioid regulation of locus coeruleus norepinephrine neurons and induces a state of cellular and physical opiate dependence. *Neuropsychopharmacology*. 2013;38:1833–1843.

28. Valentino RJ, Van Bockstaele E. Endogenous opioids: the downside of opposing stress. *Neurobiol Stress*. 2015;1:23–32.

29. Elman I, Borsook D. Common brain mechanisms of chronic pain and addiction. *Neuron*. 2016;89:11–36.

8
From causal to moral models of pain, and the right to pain relief

Introduction: the roots of opioid policies

Our opioid policies, like a right to pain relief, are based on our moral theories about responsibility for pain and opioid use. These moral theories are, in turn, based on our mechanical causal theories about the origins of pain. We have many intuitions about the mechanical causes of pain experience that fail on closer examination. We often think of pain as something that happens to us. But it is actually injuries that happen to us, and pain is something that our bodies do to protect us. We think that damage to the body produces pain in the mind or in the brain, but how does objective damage (or damage-induced nervous activity, nociception) become pain experience? We see most human suffering (e.g., depression, loneliness, rejection) as an intensely personal experience, yet we see pain as the product of an impersonal mechanical process. Only after nociception is transmitted to our brain, where it is perceived and elicits an emotional reaction, does it become personal. But this cannot explain the profound effects on pain experience produced by the interpersonal context of that experience. We have separated pain from suffering, and from the rest of human culture, and given it over to medicine to explain and control.

In this chapter, we will explore the links between our current causal and moral models of pain and explain how these provide the basis for the assertion of a right to pain relief. We argue that our causal models of pain shape our moral models of pain and, thereby, our pain and opioid policies. An unexplored feature of our modern scientific research into pain mechanisms is how this has covertly shaped our ideas about responsibility for suffering. This hidden link ties together our pain science and our opioid policy. Ending our current opioid epidemic and preventing any future opioid epidemics will require challenging the special moral status of pain as passive and innocent suffering and the mechanical model of pain causation that is its foundation.

Suzanne Harris, part 1

Suzanne Harris, a 36-year-old registered nurse, comes to your office complaining of abdominal pain that began 7 years ago, when she was 29 years old. At that time, she was diagnosed with sigmoid diverticulitis with an abscess, and she was treated with a sigmoid colectomy. She recovered well from the surgery with a healed wound, no further evidence of infection, and the return of normal gastrointestinal function.

Some 2 years after her surgery, she was unfortunately stabbed in the right lower quadrant of her abdomen by an unknown man when she was outside her apartment emptying her trash. Luckily, she had only a superficial abdominal wound requiring a couple of sutures and some bruises. But she reported severe stabbing and cramping pain in this area that disrupted her ability to work, her social activities, and her bicycle riding and tennis playing. Physical examination and a magnetic resonance imaging (MRI) scan of her abdomen and pelvis were normal except for evidence of her previous surgery.

You wonder how these different elements of Suzanne's history are related to her current pain problem.

Overview: moral and causal models of pain

Moral and causal models of pain have always been intertwined. In Chapter 1, we discussed the transition from the medieval view of pain as the proper punishment for sin, both the original sin of Adam and Eve and the sins of individuals, to the Enlightenment view of pain as a natural misfortune. Our modern medical view of pain has continued to see it as a natural event, understood more clearly in causal terms (i.e., how does pain happen?) than in moral terms (i.e., why does pain happen?). Nevertheless, an implicit moral model of pain underlies this causal model. This moral model sees pain as arising from the universal human vulnerability to death and disease, for which each of us is blameless. It is our fate, but not our fault, that we will all eventually fall ill and die. Pain is a natural part of that process and of our body's effort to avoid premature death. This means that patients with pain are not responsible for the pain that they present for care. They have done nothing to cause or deserve what they experience. This lack of responsibility for being in pain is extended to include a lack of accountability for recovery from pain. This causal passivity and its moral corollary, innocence, are the basis for the claim of a right to pain relief. Whereas medieval pain was interpreted as a sign of sin, contemporary pain tends to be interpreted as a sign of the absence of sin because it is understood as a mechanical product of impersonal forces.

This passive suffering provides the moral basis for the right to pain relief. The scientific root of this right's claim is the mechanical account of pain, which describes how pain is imposed on an innocent victim. We separate pain (as produced by impersonal mechanisms originating within the body) from suffering (as arising from personal and interpersonal meanings originating between bodies). This mechanical account of pain causation has always worked better for acute pain than chronic pain, which is why acute pain is more purely innocent. Ambiguities about causation mean that the moral status of chronic pain has been murkier. The moral argument for a right to relief of chronic pain has drawn upon earlier successful arguments for rights to relief of acute pain and pain at the end of life. But the right to pain relief is limited: It only applies, for example, to the use of prescribed opioids for the treatment of physical pain, never for the social pain arising from abandonment or abuse. Within our medical model that separates pain from the rest of human suffering, we reserve access to opioids only for medical and mechanical pain. If there is any right to treatment of social pain through psychotherapy, it is qualified by the requirement that the patient participate actively in the treatment.

In our modern era, this *moral* model of pain is based on a *causal* model of pain, which sees pain as caused by impersonal mechanisms inside the body. Tissue damage produces specific nociceptive activity in the nervous system that is transmitted from the injured body part to the brain where it is received and perceived. Descartes described the essentials of this mechanical model in 1664 (see Figure 1.3 in Chapter 1):

> If for example fire comes near the foot, minute particles of this fire, which you know to move at great velocity, have the power to set in motion the spot of skin on the foot which they touch, and by this means pulling on a delicate thread which is attached to the spot of the skin, they open up at the same instant the pore against which the delicate thread ends, just as by pulling on one end of a rope one makes to strike at the same instant a bell which hangs at the end.[1(p18)]

Descartes's model has been extensively investigated and modified in the nearly 400 years since it was proposed. It has been directly and explicitly challenged by the past 50 years of pain research. But we will argue that crucial elements of this model have been preserved, most especially the mechanical elements that support the moral model of pain as undeserved suffering. We argue that this model of pain as passive and innocent suffering must be challenged if we are to end our current opioid epidemic and prevent a future opioid epidemic.

In place of this mechanical medical model of pain, we will propose an alternative model of pain as a protective homeostatic emotion that promotes survival through a sophisticated and adaptable system of danger detection. This system detects threats to the integrity of body and person, using aversive experiences like pain, anxiety, and depression as signals for more and less immediate threats to bodily tissue. According to this homeostatic emotion theory, the person is involved in the causation and relief of pain through the interpretation and response to threats of danger. Pain is no longer seen as the product of a purely impersonal process. The causes of pain include both impersonal and personal elements, similar to the causation of anxiety and depression. This is especially true of chronic pain, which becomes intertwined with the beliefs and behaviors of the person with pain. This means that the person benefits from active participation in the care for their chronic pain, as do patients with other chronic illnesses like diabetes. It is not adequate to simply present oneself for care as a victim of chronic illness, asking the clinician to "fix me." This passive positioning of the patient has not generally provided the patient long-lasting relief, nor does it empower the patient to provide effective self-care.

Explaining pain by neurobiological mechanisms

As we have come to approach pain as a medical phenomenon over the past two centuries, there has been a vigorous effort to explain pain in terms of neurobiological mechanisms. In Kenneth Casey's excellent 2019 book *Chasing Pain: The Search for a Neurobiological Mechanism*,[2] a moral agenda is apparent from the first sentences of the introduction, entitled "Why Pain?": "No human experience is more important than physical pain. Unlike psychological pain, physical pain is experienced as an unpleasant, offensive, often threatening, and sometimes unbearable sensation on or within the body.... Death is preferred over prolonged, severe pain."[2(p1)] But since Casey's book is a modern medical account of pain, the primary questions he strives to answer are causal questions:

> What are the physical mechanisms that are directly responsible for pain? What is the biology or, more specifically, the *neuro*biology of pain? And what can the neuronal mechanisms of pain tell us about brain function generally? Pain is an experience that arises somewhere in the brain. How does this happen? Pain is a neurobiological phenomenon.[2(p2)]

Casey's statement that "pain is a neurobiological phenomenon" is factual, but he does not provide direct evidence for it. It is the assumption upon which his book is based: "We know that pain emerges from the activity of the nervous system."[2(p2)] The social and moral context within which our neurobiology operates is thought to be fully expressed and explained through that neurobiology. These are the remaining footprints of Descartes, who claimed we only need to look *inside* the body to explain pain.

Remember that the approach to pain as a medical problem, like the Enlightenment approach to pain as a social problem, is devoted to the reduction of pain to a minimum. This goal justifies the mechanical approach for Casey:

> We chase pain because we wish to control it. And we wish to control it *selectively*, without compromising or interfering with other

experiences or body functions.... But an experience cannot be seen, touched, or manipulated. To control something, we usually must understand it in a mechanistic way so that we can manipulate its component parts and determine the direction and intensity of its action or activity.[2(p2)]

The mechanical approach to pain is, thus, a pragmatic approach. But it also strives to be a complete account of pain causation: "To put it simply, *we wish to identify the structures that as a group are necessary and sufficient for pain*" (emphasis in original).[2(p3)] We will explore below how this mechanical model of pain causation has been developed through investigations into nociception, pain transmission, and perception. And despite many significant advances in pain research over the last 50 years, some of the questions that haunt Descartes's mechanical model of pain persist:

1. At what point in the nervous system is objective nociception transformed into subjective pain?
2. How are impersonal pain mechanisms transformed into the intensely personal pain experience?

Suzanne Harris, part 2

You begin thinking about Suzanne's pain as we have thought about pain for hundreds of years, in terms of the relation between a potentially damaging noxious stimulus and her pain experience. It makes sense for abdominal pain to be caused by sigmoid diverticulitis and abscess. This pain is expected to have sensory-discriminative (location, quality), cognitive-evaluative (do I have infection?, cancer?), and affective-emotional (fear, dread) dimensions. It makes sense to remove the stimulus with a colectomy. But the abdominal pain after the superficial stabbing is harder to explain in these terms.

Impersonal pain neurophysiological mechanisms

Nociception: causation and transmission of pain-specific nervous system activity

If you were studying how pain is caused by noxious stimuli like mechanical pressure, heat, or cold, it makes sense to study how noxious stimuli are detected, encoded, and transmitted in the nervous system. This is known as the study of nociception, or pain-specific activity in the nervous system. Other senses, like vision and hearing, have dedicated sensory organs and nerves in which sensory information is transmitted. Investigators thought this likely to be true of pain as well. The specificity theory of pain postulates a dedicated pain receptor leading through a dedicated pain fiber to a dedicated pain center in the brain. In 1947, Sherrington extended the specificity theory through investigation of the functional basic unit of nociception, the simple reflex arc, which added a motor component to the basic pain experience. In the late 1960s, Edward Perl reported the discovery of specific receptors (nociceptors) and fibers for nociception, which appeared to confirm a dedicated nervous system for pain perception.

In 1965, *Science* published a seminal paper by Ronald Melzack and Patrick Wall, "Pain Mechanisms: A New Theory," that described the "gate control theory of pain."[3] This theory was opposed to the idea that there were "labeled lines" with pain receptors and pain fibers as proposed in the specificity theory. It famously proposed that there was a neurological "gate" in the spinal cord that balanced inputs from small-diameter (noxious stimulus sensing) and large-diameter (touch sensing) fibers before relaying nociceptive information up the spinothalamic tract to the brain. It also proposed that this relay process was modulated by a descending "central control" function that was not well specified at that time. The gate control theory opened the modern era of pain research that sees pain as continuously modulated by the nervous system to optimize the organism's response to its overall situation.

At the time of the famous 1973 Bonica-convened meeting in Issaquah, Washington, the pain field was torn between the specificity theory and the gate control theory of pain. Kenneth Casey summarizes the state of the science at that time:

The terms "nociceptor" and "gate control" could be considered opposing ends of a spectrum of ideas about pain at the Issaquah meeting.
.... The term "nociceptor" conjures in the causal mind the concept that
pain is inextricably linked to a fully deterministic peripheral sensory
apparatus. Thus, there are "pain receptors" and "pain fibers" ... The
concept of "gate control" tends to dissociate pain from the activation
of peripheral nociceptors by emphasizing that a complex neurophysiology underlies pain and that the [central nervous system, CNS] controls sensation.[2(p19)]

This debate between specificity and pattern theories has continued to the
present day, with most investigators accepting that specific nociceptive
receptors and fibers dominate in the peripheral nervous system while complex pattern recognition by multifunction neurons and centers dominates
in the CNS.[4] The consensus among pain researchers has only been partially
absorbed by clinicians, who still generally consider pain to be a symptom of
bodily damage that is transmitted to the patient's brain, where it is experienced and then presented for clinical care.

To definitively break with the standard passive, mechanical model of pain
perception, we must reject the idea that perception is something that happens
to us or in us; rather, it is something we do. Bodies are injured by external
forces, but pain is a protective experience produced by the body and brain.
Pain is not part of the passive injury process, but part of the active protection process. In his *Action in Perception*, philosopher Alva Noe has taken this
notion further by arguing that "perceiving is a way of acting."[5] Perception,
including pain perception, is a form of action that the organism uses to survive in the world. "*What we perceive* is determined by *what we do* (or what we
know how to do); it is determined by what we are *ready* to do."[5(p85)] Pain is not
something that happens to an organism. It is something that the organism
does to protect itself. It is, in essence, a command to protect oneself.

Suzanne Harris, part 3

Suzanne's abdominal pain is more than her diverticulitis. Somehow her
abdominal pain got worse after a minor stabbing injury that did not

penetrate her abdominal wall. Although her diverticulitis was more visible on imaging than any cause of her current pain, she says her pain is
worse now, after her diverticulitis has resolved. She is puzzled and trou-
bled by this. If her bowel is OK, why does it feel as if it is not OK? A more
complex understanding of Suzanne's pain perception is needed if you are
going to be able to explain how the superficial stabbing produced such severe and prolonged pain for Suzanne.

Studying pain perception: where and how does nociception become pain?

In our standard understanding of pain perception, the work of nociception
is assigned to the peripheral nervous system, the work of pain perception
to the CNS. Noxious stimuli are encoded by nociceptors, and nociceptive
information is transmitted to the spinal cord, from which it is conveyed to
the brain. This idea of nociceptive transmission led to many attempts by
neurosurgeons to provide lasting relief from intractable pain by interrupting
this transmission. Cutting procedures have taken many forms over the past
century, such as neurectomies (where peripheral nerves are cut), spinothalamic tractotomies (where the ascending spinal cord tract is cut), dorsal root
entry zone lesions (where the entry point of the sensory dorsal root into the
cord is lesioned), cordotomies (where the cord is transected wholly or partially), thalamotomies (lesioning the thalamus where the spinothalamic tract
enters), gyrectomies (involving resection of a cortical gyrus), and finally prefrontal lobotomies (where connection to the prefrontal cortex is severed)
(Figure 8.1).

These procedures to interrupt nociception have largely been abandoned (except for patients with a short life span) because they do not
provide lasting and reliable pain relief. They have different effects
depending on the level at which the neurons are damaged. But an initial period of numbness is often followed by an enduring sensitive and
painful body part. The failure of these procedures throws into doubt our
ideas about nociceptive information transmission and even our ideas
about the functional localization of pain in the nervous system. As Casey
has summarized:

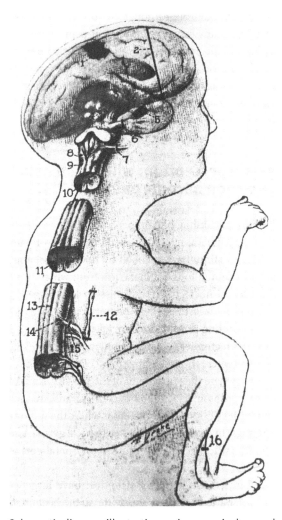

Figure 8.1. Schematic diagram illustrating various surgical procedures designed to alleviate pain

In summary, the attempt to provide a lasting and selective relief from pain by destroying parts of the CNS is disappointing.... Thus, the concept of functional localization of pain in the nervous system is brought into question. There does not appear to be a single, completely private CNS pathway for pain—a structure or pathway that has this function and no other. This raises the question of what is meant by "functional localization." How is function defined? And at what anatomical or structural level is location within the CNS defined? Are there single or multiple points and pathways?[2(p30)]

This failure to relieve pain by interrupting transmission also raises the question as to whether our ideas about the separation of nociceptive transmission from pain perception are correct. One way in which this question has been taken up by philosophers is to ask: After I bash my thumb with a hammer, is it more correct to say that the pain is in my hand or that the pain is in my brain?[6] If pain is a perceptual object, it makes sense to say the pain is in my hand. If pain is a subjective experience, then it makes more sense to say that the pain is in my brain. In a famous story, the philosopher Bertrand Russell was asked by his dentist, "Where does it hurt?" "In my mind, of course," Russell replied. This was stated 100 years ago, and it echoes a statement made by Descartes nearly 300 years before Russell: "Pain in the hand is felt by the soul not because the soul is present in the hand but because the soul is present in the brain." A modern Russell would reply to his dentist, "In my brain, of course," for we no longer believe in a soul behind or beyond the brain. If pain is understood as a sensation (or a representation of tissue damage) produced in the periphery and perceived in the brain, it is essentially a private illusion. As Ramachandran and Blakeslee stated in their 1998 book on the brain, "Pain itself is an illusion—constructed entirely in your brain like any other sensory experience."[7(p58)] This "pain as illusion" is the odd, clinically unhelpful, corner we are backed into by our usual causal account of pain, where nociception is generated in the periphery and then transmitted to the brain, where it is perceived.

It is certainly true that a functioning brain is necessary for the perception of pain. But to say that pain perception occurs within the brain is to make a more specific and contentious claim: that the process of nociception becomes suddenly self-aware at some point in the brain. Yet it has been difficult to determine which brain centers are necessary and sufficient for the perception of pain—or how these brain centers turn nociception into pain.

Descartes understood the nervous system, including the brain, as a mechanical operation. But as a mechanical operation, it could not perceive or know anything. For Descartes, these "knowing" functions were part of the immaterial mind, which communicated with the brain through the pineal gland. We now reject Descartes's dualism out of hand, believing that there is no immaterial *res cogitans* mind lurking above or beyond the brain. There is *only* the brain. So, we think, this brain *must* be where pain perception occurs. But there is a serious problem with this commonsense view. If nociceptive information is transmitted from the periphery to the center where it is perceived as pain, where is this center? This center has been named the pain matrix and usually includes the thalamus, somatosensory cortex, cingulate gyrus, and insula, among other centers. But the difficult question is: How do these brain centers turn nociception into pain? The more specific difficult question is: How do we get from nociceptive transmission to pain perception?

Among the many philosophers who have tried to answer this question, Daniel Dennett argued that Cartesian materialism necessarily implies that there is a crucial "finish line" somewhere in the brain where the brain becomes conscious of itself. This is the center at which nociceptive transmission ends and pain perception begins. Dennett calls this the Cartesian theater, where a small version of ourselves (a homunculus) might be watching a movie produced by our brains (Figure 8.2).[8] Silly and childish? Perhaps, but any attempt to explain how transmission becomes perception runs into this problem.

There is, of course, no little man inside us who watches the movie produced by our visual system, nor a little man who feels the pain produced by our somatosensory system. There is, in fact, no point in our nervous system where nociception (objective nervous system activity) turns into pain (subjective experience). Philosopher and psychiatrist Thomas Fuchs explains:

> Where is the pain now when my foot hurts me? According to the common neuroscientific belief, it is where it is produced, that is, in the brain ... However, the brain does not feel pains, nor does it contain them ...

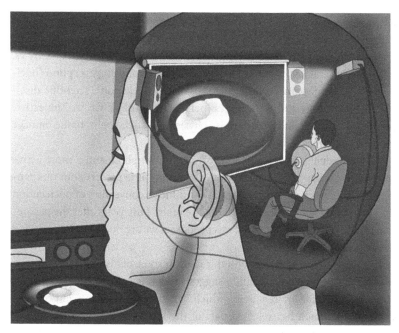

Figure 8.2. Cartesian theater from Dennett. A tiny person sits in a movie theater inside a human head, watching and hearing and feeling everything that is being experienced by the human being.

https://commons.wikimedia.org/wiki/File:Cartesian_Theater.svg. Derivative work: Pbroks13Original: Jennifer Garcia (Reverie), CC BY-SA 2.5 <https://creativecommons.org/licenses/by-sa/2.5>, via Wikimedia Commons

The pain-in-the-foot is thus *neither* in the physical space of the foot, *nor* is it in the physical space of the brain, for pains are, after all, neither anatomical things such as sinews, bones or neurons, nor are they physiological processes such as charge-transfers at neuronal cell membranes. Where is the pain then? It is in the "foot as part of the living body" for this unified living body also produces—not least by means of the brain—*a spatially extended body subjectivity.*[9(p16)]

Modern pain clinicians and scientists vehemently reject Cartesian dualism as unscientific. We scoff at the idea of an immaterial mind perceiving pain. But we replicate this dualism all the time when explaining pain perception as a two-step process, with a passive receptive phase in the body followed by an active interpretive phase in the brain. We resort to a wide variety of dualistic concepts in our pain explanations, which can refer to body parts (body vs. brain, peripheral nervous system vs. CNS), phases of pain perception (nociception vs. pain, pain vs. suffering, sensation vs. reaction), scientific disciplines (physiology vs. psychology), perspectives (objective vs. subjective, public vs. private), and pain causes (physical vs. social pain, tissue damage vs. personal threat) (Table 8.1).

All these dualisms separate a passive receptive phase and a more active interpretive phase in pain perception. They allow us to preserve our mechanical model of nociception by pushing the difficult conversion of nociception into pain into some obscure corner of the brain. Fifty years after the perceptive function of the pain matrix was proposed, we are no closer to clarifying its mysterious mechanism.

Patrick Wall has grappled with this issue in some of his writings: "[E]very aspect of our conscious sensation suggests that it is not fed by a passive machine but includes brain activity, which has directed attention and ordered exploration, which has selected part of the sensory input and has amplified information about details.[1(p24)] Later in his book *Pain: The Science of Suffering*, Wall elaborates on this "active participation of mind and body":

> We naturally think in steps. First we have sensation, followed by perception with its identification, classification, and emotion, and last, perhaps, motor action and behavior.... *Could it be that we have made*

Table 8.1 Remnants of dualism in pain science

Pain dualisms	Passive receptive	Active interpretive
Body parts	Body Peripheral nervous system	Brain CNS
Pain perception phases	Nociception Pain sensation	Pain perception Emotional reaction, suffering
Scientific disciplines	Physiology	Psychology, sociology
Perspectives	Objective Public	Subjective Private
Pain causes	Physical damage	Social damage

a fundamental error in expecting a sensory box separate from the motor-planning box? Could it be that we in fact sense objects in terms of what we might do about them? Could it be that we have erected an artificial frontier between a sensory brain and a motor-planning brain that does not in fact exist?[1(p57)]

Wall is suggesting that to solve the dualism of mind and body in pain may mean questioning the dualism of the sensory and motor systems. It may mean rejecting the idea of pain perception as a passive reception of information about tissue damage.

Wall approaches the insight of philosopher Alva Noe that "[p]erception is not something that happens to us, or in us. It is something we do."[5(p92)] Pain makes sense only as a survival strategy of the organism. It is not a show put on for us by the brain. Noe argues that "we ought to reject the idea—widespread in both philosophy and science—that perception is a process *in the brain* whereby the perceptual system constructs an *internal representation* of the world." Pain is not a representation of tissue damage; it exists because it informs action. "*What we perceive* is determined by *what we do* (or what we know how to do); it is determined by what we are *ready* to do." Sensory experiences don't just inform motor behavior, they are shaped by our capacities for motor behavior. Here, Noe goes beyond Wall's argument, for he "proposes not that perceiving is *for* acting, but rather that perceiving is constituted by the exercise of a range of sensorimotor skills." If reflex withdrawal is the only motor option available, sensory pain experience only needs to determine whether reflex withdrawal is appropriate or not. If more complex motor options are available, more complex sensory discriminations are needed: "[W]hen we perceive, we perceive in an idiom of possibilities for movement." If we are only capable of reflex withdrawal, pain needs only turn this reflex on. But if we can scream and limp and seek help and file disability claims, the pain experience needs to be richer and more flexible.

Noe argues that "to perceive you must have sensory stimulation that *you understand.*"[(p93)] By understanding, he means a sensorimotor understanding: What am I to do with this information? If pain is a sensorimotor protective action, it is no longer a passive reception of noxious stimuli. Pain is not an apprehension or representation of tissue damage, but a call to action.

Suzanne Harris, part 4

Searching for an explanation of her abdominal pain after her superficial stabbing, you ask Suzanne for more details of that experience. She explains that at the time of her stabbing, she was in the middle of a difficult divorce that followed the loss of a pregnancy a year before. There was some question of whether her estranged husband had tried to exact revenge by attacking her, but he claimed to be across town that evening and had witnesses who corroborated this alibi.

Suzanne denies earlier trauma in her life, including any childhood abuse or neglect. However, she has almost no memory of her high school years, during which her parents went through an angry and prolonged divorce. In addition to constant abdominal pain since the stabbing, Suzanne reports nightmares of being stabbed and being very "jumpy," with an increased startle response to any surprise. She avoids any reminders of the evening when her stabbing occurred and won't put out the trash after dark. She is not interested in seeing friends or exploring any new romantic relationships, though her friends have tried to introduce her to eligible men.

What is perceived when we experience pain: damage or danger?

As Casey states, we investigate pain in order to control it, seeking to identify unique molecular mechanisms, receptors, pathways, and brain centers for pain so we can target these with therapies. He identifies this as one pragmatic reason for the lasting appeal of at least some version of the specificity theory that postulates unique pathways and centers for pain perception. It has long been apparent that pain is not perceived in one specific brain center. Brain lesions that affect pain also affect other neurological functions. For example, small lesions in the thalamus produce not only loss of pain and temperature sensation, but also loss of tactile, vibratory, and kinesthetic sensations.

Multiple authors argue that what was formerly called the "pain matrix" of brain centers specific to pain perception is more properly considered a multisensory "salience network,"[10-12] activated by sensory events of various modalities that indicate a threat to the body's integrity. These events include not only nociceptive stimuli, but also non-nociceptive stimuli (e.g., visual, auditory) that determine the salience or relevance of nociception to organism survival. Non-nociceptive sensory stimuli, if salient, may produce a pattern of brain activity virtually identical to that produced by nociceptive stimuli.[13] Visual information of approaching threats can increase nociceptive responses in somatosensory centers. Therefore, the activity in the brain areas that respond to nociceptive stimuli is a reflection not of pain intensity, but of pain salience. Stimuli that are more intense are generally more salient. Intensity has been favored as the most important feature of noxious stimuli because intensity is an objective property of the stimulus. According to psychophysical experiments, this stimulus intensity was mirrored in the intensity of the pain experience. But these were controlled experiments, not actually threatening clinical situations. Threat and salience cannot be studied with psychophysical techniques. Salience is *not* an objective property of the stimulus; rather, it is a measure of the importance of the stimulus for the organism and its survival. In moving from stimulus *intensity* to stimulus *salience*, we have thus begun to move from a primacy of *mechanism* to a primacy of *meaning* in pain causation.

The brain salience network expands the influences on pain experience from nociception to multisensory indicators of safety or danger, and thus offers the means for personal meaning (specifically the relevance to survival) to interact with impersonal nociceptive mechanisms. According to Legrain and colleagues: "Indeed, salience detectors represent neural mechanisms by which selective attention is captured and oriented towards the most salient stimuli in order to prioritize their processing over background stimuli, to improve their perception and to prompt appropriate action."[12(p15)] The central role played by salience in pain perception means "that the purpose of pain is not merely to induce and to associate the feeling of unpleasantness to a somatosensory sensation, but it also to warn the body about potential physical threats." This salience detection system will react to a wasp approaching my hand even before it actually stings my hand.

Thus, this detection of threats is not limited to damage within the body. Legrain and colleagues explains, "Responding adequately to events that threaten the body's integrity constitutes an action whose achievement requires close interaction with systems that are able to localize threatening information in the proximal space of the body."[12(p120)] Salience network neurons may respond to visual objects when they are *approaching* the body, but not when they are *moving away* from the body. Salience detection includes the "peripersonal space," which includes the body *and* the environment within grasping distance. There is a close relationship between visual, proprioceptive, and tactile processing of threats in this peripersonal space.

In fact, salience offers a means of synthesizing many physiological and psychological processes—or mechanical and meaningful influences—on pain perception. For example, brain hyperactivation in response to pain onset and offset in fibromyalgia patients has been interpreted as evidence of "aberrant salience."[14] This consists of aberrant functioning of the brain circuits that assign salience values to stimuli and may contribute to chronic pain. According to Borsook and colleagues, the salience network helps explain "feeling pain in the absence of a painful stimulus, reporting minimal pain in the setting of major trauma, having an 'analgesic' response in the absence of an active treatment, or reporting no pain relief after administration of a potent analgesic."[11(p100)] The salience idea thus accounts for much of the puzzling mismatch between the amount of tissue damage sustained and the amount of pain experienced, such as we have seen in the case of Suzanne. The salience network, centered on the anterior insula, integrates sensory, emotional, and cognitive information to determine reward, motivation, and emotion. It couples the anterior insula with the dorsal anterior cingulate cortex to regulate avoidance motor behavior. The salience network thus offers the means of integrating pain with other negative, protective experiences like anxiety and depression.[15]

As we mentioned in Chapter 5, Lorimer Moseley and David Butler from Australia have incorporated these insights about pain salience into their Explaining Pain (EP) program for treating chronic pain. The central insight transmitted to patients by the EP program is that the pain system is not a tissue *damage* detection system; rather, it is a tissue *danger* detection system. *While damage can be detected on physical examination and MRI scans, danger cannot.* Moseley and Butler argue that "pain is fundamentally dependent on meaning" because it "reflects an implicit evaluation of danger to body tissue and the need for protective behavior."[18(p810)] Moseley and Butler is opposed to the idea that acute pain is nociceptive, while much of chronic pain is not. Because he conceives of the pain system as protecting against danger, not just damage, he does not distinguish between eudynia (helpful acute pain) and maldynia (unhelpful chronic pain).[16] EP sees all clinical pain as cognitively modulated. This modulation is not limited to chronic pain; it affects not just the interpretation of pain, but its intensity. They explain:

> When pain persists and feels like it is ruining your life, it is difficult to see how it can be serving any useful purpose. But even when pain is chronic and nasty, it hurts because the brain has concluded, for some reason or another, that you are threatened and in danger and need protecting—the trick is finding out why the brain has come to this conclusion.[17(p11)]

The therapeutic focus is to reduce the threat value of movement and living in order to reduce pain. "EP emphasizes that any credible evidence of danger to body tissue can increase pain and any credible evidence of safety to body tissue can decrease pain."[18(p809)]

Most importantly, this meaning-centered model of pain has provided the basis for an effective pain treatment program. Unlike cognitive–behavioral therapy (CBT) and other forms of pain psychology, EP does not focus on coping or managing the patient's pain experience. It does not aim to change the patient's reaction to pain or to mitigate pain-related suffering. It aims to reduce the pain itself. Rather than helping patients "live well with pain," it seeks to help them "live well without pain." EP aims to "change someone's understanding of the biological processes of pain as a mechanism to reduce pain itself."[(p808)] In a 12-month study, an improvement in pain biology knowledge was significantly associated with a reduction in pain intensity and an improvement in function over time.[19] Use of EP in a wide variety of formats has been proven to improve patients' pain and reduce disability when added to other programs that aim to increase mobility and exercise.[20] Key messages in the EP program include the variable relationship between nociception and pain, the potent influence of context on pain, up-regulation in the danger detection system as pain persists, the fact that pain is influenced by several interacting protective systems, and, above all, the adaptability and trainability of our pain biology.

The EP approach contrasts with the recent assertion that chronic pain is a brain disease independent of the person's attitudes and behaviors. EP does not focus on any pathological pain generator, whether in the peripheral nervous system (e.g., nociception driving central sensitization) or in the CNS (e.g., chronic pain as brain disease). EP targets the faulty threat/safety discrimination in patients with chronic pain. It does this through a program of neuroscience-based pain education. EP works on its own, but works best as part of a comprehensive biopsychosocial rehabilitation effort.[21] Such an effort combines didactic learning in the classroom with experiential learning using body movement and relaxation techniques. The EP program provides evidence that the new conceptualization of pain within the homeostatic emotion framework of salience and danger detection can advance chronic pain treatment as well as theory.

What role for nociception? What is its purpose and meaning?

Activation of nociceptors and nociceptive pathways by noxious stimuli can give rise to pain. This helps us protect our tissues from injury. But neuroscientists Baliki and Apkarian remind us that nociception usually protects us *before* prompting the conscious experience of pain.[22] I don't damage myself by sitting completely immobile for hours while I write this, because I shift and squirm unconsciously in my chair. We don't injure ourselves when walking or grasping things—as do those with syphilis or leprosy—because we modulate our activity before we injure ourselves and before we feel pain. Most peripheral nociceptors can be activated by stimuli that are subthreshold for pain. "As a result, the nociceptive control of behavior routinely occurs in the absence of consciously perceived pain, rendering it 'subconscious.'"[22(p480)] Whether nociception is perceived as pain depends on many salience-related factors beyond the intensity of the nociception. Much of the time, nociception can do its work protecting tissue without disrupting our ongoing mental processes with the experience of pain. But if the nociception is too intense *or if the situation is otherwise judged to be significantly threatening*, pain is produced by the organism to protect itself from harm.

Baliki and Apkarian have proposed that pain perception, as distinct from nociception, is part of a continuum of aversive behavioral learning that is manifested by pain, anxiety, or depression, depending on preexisting vulnerabilities.[22] They envisage pain and negative moods as a continuum of aversive behavioral learning, which enhances survival by protecting against threats. Threats that are most immediate in time and in space are experienced as pain. Those that are somewhat less immediate and less localized to a body part are experienced as anxiety. Those that are yet more global and enduring are experienced as depression. In this way, the Baliki and Apkarian framework for the transformation of nociception into behavior selection through learning is extended to incorporate negative moods.[23] They reject the idea that pain is a mechanically produced sensation and that anxiety and depression are emotional reactions.

We think of pain and pleasure as feelings, long considered opposites. Yet the feelings of pain and pleasure cannot be understood in isolation from the organism's and the species' quest for survival. Pain is not just a feeling, but also a behavioral drive.[24] As Porreca and Navratilova have recently written, "Pain is a call to action. Like hunger, thirst, and desire for sleep, pain is a part of the body's survival systems that collectively are responsible for protecting the organism."[25(pS45)] This emotional-drive aspect of pain has been recognized since 1968 when Melzack and Casey replaced a purely sensory model of pain with a multidimensional model that recognized not only sensory/discriminative aspect of pain but also affective/motivational features.[26] Recognition of the affective dimension of pain is now widespread, but the idea that the sensory dimension is *subordinated* to the affective dimension is more novel. The affective apparatus of the limbic system dampens or amplifies the pain experience according to the overall situation of the organism. What is actually felt, be it perceived pain or pleasure, is the product of calculation within the mesolimbic reward systems, which aligns nociceptive processing with reward to promote survival of the organism. Pain has survival value because it has action implications.

Pain is primarily imperative rather than informative

The focus on pain's role in our survival represents a fundamental reconception of pain. Since Descartes, we have considered pain to be a sensory experience that represents the state of our body for our mind. Pain's function, on the Cartesian view, is to provide information about the world that is outside our mind. Specifically, it provides information about damage to our body. But what if these standard views of pain's function are seriously mistaken? In *What the Body Commands: The Imperative Theory of Pain*, philosopher Colin Klein argues that "[a]ll pains have imperative content, and that imperative content is what distinguishes them as pains."[27(p1)] An imperative is a command, not a representation or a description. Klein argues that the primary function of pain is to *command* protective behavior rather than to *inform* us of tissue damage. This may seem like a trivial or nitpicking distinction, but it is not.

Most sensory experiences, such as visual and auditory (olfaction may be an exception[28]), inform us of the outside world, but pain does not. "Ordinary sensations inform but don't necessarily motivate. Pains motivate without informing. That is why pain is unusual."[27(p3)] Visual sensory experience provides us information about the world that can be determined to be either true or false: Was that really a ghost or just a sheet flapping in the breeze? Is that my mother calling my name or someone else? But pains are not true or false in the usual sense of correspondence with reality. Commands are not true and false in this usual sense: "What is commanded is to be *made* true." A patient or clinician can investigate the cause of pain, but this does not prove the experience of pain to be a true or false representation. Clinicians often consider pains without clear association with tissue damage as "false" or as unreal pain or non-medical pain. But this assumes that real pain is caused by tissue damage. But modern pain research has revealed the relationship between pain and tissue damage to be loose, variable, and continuously modified, as reviewed above. If pain arises from danger detection, its truth or falsity is more complicated. There is no simple division between real pain associated with visible damage and unreal or exaggerated pain not associated with visible damage. Danger is not an objective property of the body.

According to this view, pain represents not the state of the external world but rather the state of the internal world of our body. Neuroscientist Bud Craig first argued that pain is an interoceptive (internally focused) faculty, not an exteroceptive (externally focused) faculty. He thus referred to pain as a "homeostatic emotion."[24] Pain is processed in the body like temperature, not like vision or audition, and like our temperature sense, pain tells us about the integrity of the body. It asks: Is homeostasis threatened? Klein explains, "The biological role of pain is a homeostatic one. Like hunger or thirst, pain is there to get you to act in ways that bring your body back into balance."[27(p3)] Pain exists to get you to do something protective. Pain does have sensory features like location and quality (aching, pricking), but these are often imprecise and exist to serve pain's primary protective function.

The link between pain and protection helps explain the variable relationship between pain and tissue damage. "Painless injury occurs ... precisely when such protective actions would be maladaptive by prohibiting the necessary avoidance of dangerous situations. When safety should take priority over protection, injury may end up painless."[27(p32)] A classic example of painless injury occurs when an animal is injured while fleeing a predator. The animal's endogenous opioid system suppresses pain until the animal is safe from the predator and protection of the injured body part again becomes most important for survival.[29] Patrick Wall argues that this delayed persistent pain, which promotes rest and recuperation, may be more important for survival than the initial pain that motivates withdrawal from the noxious stimulus. As Wall stated in 1979, "Pain is a poor protector against injury since it occurs far too late in the case of sudden injury or of very slow damage to provide a useful preventive measure. Instead it is proposed that pain signals the existence of a body state where recovery and recuperation should be initiated."[27(p29)]

This delayed protective pain can persist when safety has not been restored. The traditional distinction between acute and chronic pain relies on the idea of tissue healing time. On the traditional view of pain as a sign of tissue damage, when the tissue damage has healed, pain should cease. According to Bonica, chronic pain is pain that persists beyond healing time.[30] But the imperative, danger-focused pain theory offers an alternative understanding. Pain persists when danger to integrity persists. This can occur due to properties of the body (e.g., persistent inflammation), the person (e.g., history of psychological trauma), or the situation (e.g., ongoing threat of domestic violence). As we have seen in the case of Suzanne, danger takes many forms and its perception cannot be understood in purely mechanical terms.

The core message for us from Klein's book is that pain is more about action than information. Pain commands protective action. It is informative (e.g., about location or type of injuring agent) only insofar as that is necessary for effective protective action. Pain not only prompts protective movement (e.g., withdrawing from a flame, avoiding weight bearing on a fractured leg), but it also can itself be understood as a form of protective action. Pain is not imposed on the body; rather, it is something the body does to protect itself. Injury may happen to an animal, but pain is something the animal produces to survive.

Our belief that both injury and pain are inflicted upon us is so strong that it is difficult to give up the idea of pain perception as a passive sensory process. Over a century ago, American pragmatist philosopher John Dewey argued that perception does not begin with the sensory stimulus, but with a "sensorimotor coordination," an exploration of the environment that includes bodily movement. Thomas Fuchs quotes Dewey: "In a certain sense it is the movement, which is primary, and the sensation which is secondary, the movement of the body, head and eye muscles determining what is experienced. In other words, the real beginning is with the activity of seeing: it is looking, and not a sensation of light."[9(p130)] Our capacity to move our head and our eyes helps us distinguish between visual appearance and visual reality. It helps us determine whether a visual object is small and near to us or large and far from us. Movement is even more important for the senses of touch and pain. "Touch acquires content through movement. Touch is intrinsically active."[5(p124)] The exact same heat stimulus to the hand produces more pain if the hand is moving toward the center of the body (more threatening) than if it is moving away from the body (less threatening). This effect is stronger if I am moving my own hand than if another is moving it for me. Indeed, movement appears to have a stronger effect on the perception of noxious stimuli than tactile stimuli. These movement effects on perception are seen in chronic pain as well as acute pain.[31]

If protective movement is the most important part of pain for survival, why do we have an elaborate and rich pain experience? Why aren't withdrawal reflexes enough? In simple invertebrate organisms, noxious stimuli evoke an immediate reflex withdrawal. We don't know if these organisms have a subjective pain experience, but if they do, it is likely much simpler than ours.[32] Reflex withdrawal can also occur in more complex vertebrate organisms, but it may not. This is an important adaptive advantage. More complex organisms have the capacity to inhibit and delay a reflex response to a noxious stimulus. As Fuchs explains, "It is this inhibition and delay which opens up the space and time span for consciousness to emerge."[9] Subjectivity bridges the gap between perception and action, allowing for more complex self-protective actions to be executed. We can suppress withdrawal to execute a more effective escape or to solicit help in managing our injury. Pain experience specifically expands the space and time between noxious stimulus and response, allowing for the influence of context on protective behavior: Is life threatened? Is assistance available? This gives us more flexibility and freedom in our response to noxious stimuli and in our quest for self-preservation. "The more pronounced the inhibition is against immediate reaction, and the longer the delay between a particular need and its satisfaction, the greater become the degrees of freedom."[9(p92)] Although pain experience commands protective action, it actually provides for more flexible and adaptive action than the reflex response that it largely replaces. The multimodal pain experience is supported by the multisensory salience matrix in the brain. Both increase the flexibility and value of the pain experience to the organism in its struggle to survive and reproduce.

Our mammalian pain system is more clever than the hard-wired labeled lines proposed by specificity theory. It is even more clever than the pain matrix theory that proposed a network of dedicated somatosensory centers in the brain. Our pain system utilizes a "salience network" that allows nociception to be integrated with information from other sensory modalities. Nociception may or may not lead to pain, depending on whether the pain experience helps promote survival. Pain is thus something done by the organism that flexibly promotes protective action to preserve internal homeostatic integrity. As Klein explains:

> Homeostatic sensations thus represent a halfway house between mere reflexes and full agential desires: although they motivate action, they do so in a way that allows for deliberation and other sorts of top-down control.... Homeostatic sensations give just the right amount of flexibility: flexibility as to *when* the homeostatic demand is satisfied and *how* you satisfy it, but not as to *whether* you act or *what* you do to satisfy it.[27(p17)]

Our pain responses fall between simple involuntary reflexes and fully voluntary intentional action. We can suppress our pain-driven impulses to limp or rub the elbow we bumped, but we are hard pressed to avoid withdrawing our hand after it touches the red-hot burner on the stove. This is one source of the moral complexity of pain. Pain behavior is neither fully involuntary nor fully voluntary. It is not just a reflex, nor is it fully intentional action.

Rather than characterizing pain as a sensory process followed by a motor process, it is most accurate to characterize it as a "sense-making" process. Pain perception is not simply representing or reproducing states of the body or of the world, but also preparing for and executing actions. Pain perception is one way we make sense of the world and our place in it by determining what is salient. Pain perception is part of the process of distinguishing "favorable and unfavorable circumstances in the environment, resulting in suitable, self-preserving actions."[9(p86)] The homeostatic emotions of pain and fear "are specific psychic manifestations of self-preservation and demarcation against an intervening world."[9(p91)]

Suzanne Harris, part 5

Prior to coming to see you, Suzanne had received treatment for her pain and anxiety in the form of oxycodone (total 35 mg per day) and alprazolam 1 mg at bedtime. But she continues to have severe abdominal pain and anxiety, including regular nightmares of being stabbed. On the advice of a consulting psychiatrist, you begin treatment with prazosin, an old alpha-blocker antihypertensive medication that decreases the brain's adrenergic output. You explain to Suzanne that it should help shut off her brain's "fight-or-flight alarm" that has been going off since she was stabbed. Indeed, as the dose of prazosin is increased from 2 mg to 4 mg to 6 mg, her nightmares gradually become less violent and then disappear. She also felt less anxious and angry during the day. But she still feels afraid and shut down and uninterested in friends or romance. She still has abdominal pain, though it dominates her life less, allowing her to return to some yoga.

A biopsychosocio-action theory of pain: reuniting the "how" and "why" of pain explanation

Danger unifies biological, psychological, and social causes of chronic pain

Patients who come to the clinic for medical care of their chronic pain live in fear of being told that "it is all in your head." It is not clear whether many patients are actually told this by clinicians, but they fear it as a statement of dismissal. Its meaning is not precise. At its worst, it means there is no real pain and no legitimate claim to medical care. In this crudest formulation,

Table 8.2 Summary of transition from mechanical to survival-focused pain principles

Date	Principle	Attributed to
1660s	Pain transmitted along line-labeled system from body to mind. Separation of mind and body.	Descartes
19th–20th centuries	Identification of function- specific receptors. <u>Specificity theory</u> prevalent, along with <u>pattern theory</u> and <u>intensity theory</u>	Sherrington, Von Frey
1960s–1970s	Era of <u>psychophysics</u>, deriving rules relating objective stimulus to subjective experience of pain. Criticized for the artificiality of the experimental model and its inability to account for personal threat. Multidimensional pain theory that <u>sensory-discriminative, cognitive-evaluative, and affective-emotional dimensions exist simultaneously</u>.	Price, Melzack, Casey
1965	<u>Gate control theory</u> of pain. First suggestion that nociception was modified as it was transmitted to the brain.	Melzack and Wall
1980s–1990s	Melzack proposes concept of the <u>neuromatrix</u>, a widespread ensemble of neurons integrating both nociceptive and non-nociceptive input to produce felt sense of whole body. Modified to <u>pain matrix</u>, implying a specific pain-processing network in the brain. Some specify different brain centers for different pain dimensions. Functional brain neuroimaging cited to support notion of chronic pain as brain disease.	Melzack, Bushnell, Tracey
2000s–2010s	Proposal of a multisensory <u>"saliency" matrix</u>, including many of the pain matrix's key regions. Protective action is now believed to depend more on pain's salience than its intensity. These actions are more broadly concerned with survival than with simple withdrawal.	Legrain, Ianetti, Moureaux

(continued)

Table 8.2 Continued

Date	Principle	Attributed to
2010s–2020s	Pain, reward, and emotion are combined to support protective learning. Sensory experience does not simply inform motor behavior, but is also shaped by capacities for motor behavior. Pain arises from a danger detection system rather than a damage detection system. Pain is seen as an interoceptive "homeostatic emotion." Processed like temperature, pain informs about the integrity of the body, triggering action if the integrity of the body is threatened. Pain, including chronic pain, helps maintain a safe physical and social existence for humans.	Apkarian, Baliki, Porreca, Davis, Kucyi, Borsook, Moseley, Klein, Craig

"it is all in your head" does not distinguish between feigned pain, imagined pain, or psychological distress misinterpreted as pain. Patients rightly feel dismissed and discounted by the intimation that their pain is not legitimate, or not even real. They leave angry and frustrated.

A slightly less crude, but more common, scenario occurs when physical examination and medical imaging fail to reveal tissue damage or injury within the body that is causing the patient's chronic pain. The clinician may innocently declare, "I don't see anything on your MRI that would cause this pain." Or, if the clinician is a specialist, she may declare, "There is nothing that I can do to help you with your pain," meaning that there is no orthopedic procedure or neurological diagnosis to deploy. This conclusion may only mean that this is the wrong specialist to approach for pain relief. It is more difficult for the patient if his primary care doctor says, "There is nothing for me to do for your pain." This feels like a wholesale dismissal of one's pain from the medical world.

More common in recent years is the clinician's suggestion that his patient should go see a psychologist rather than a surgeon about his back pain problem. The patient recoils at the suggestion that the cause of the problem lies in his head rather than in his back. The standard reply at this point is to deny that the psychologist is going to see causes of the pain "deep in the patient's psyche" and to explain that the psychologist will help the patient cope more productively with the pain, thereby reducing the associated suffering and disability, if not the pain itself. Psychological intervention can also be justified by pointing to "individual differences" in pain experience for people with similar disease or injury severity.[33] Here, psychological explanation and therapy pick up where medical explanation and therapy leave off. Psychology thus addresses the "mosaic that makes pain personal."

Pain psychology has also been deployed to help explain why pain persists into chronicity.[34] The fear-avoidance model, which postulates "an interacting, cyclical sequence of fear-related cognitive, affective and behavioral processes,"[34(pT75)] successfully predicts that individuals with chronic pain and high fear-avoidance will have more pain and disability and lower return-to-work rates after treatment. There is a dose-response effect, with higher levels of fear-avoidance leading to higher likelihood of prolonged pain and disability. In fact, overall emotional distress (including depression and anxiety) predicts pain outcomes such as disability, healthcare costs, mortality, and suicide more reliably than pain intensity. Healthy individuals with more depressed mood had heightened sensitivity to experimental pain that was moderated by activity in brain areas involved in the evaluation of pain (ventrolateral prefrontal cortex, anterior insula).[35] Strong prospective links have also been demonstrated between early traumatic experiences and the development of chronic pain. Childhood physical, sexual, and emotional abuse increase the likelihood of many adult chronic pain conditions, including fibromyalgia, irritable bowel syndrome, chronic pelvic pain, and temporomandibular disorders. Past trauma increases chronic pain risk two- to three-fold. Repeated trauma especially increases the risk of chronic pain. Posttraumatic stress disorder is strongly associated with the transition from acute to chronic pain and with the severity of chronic pain once it develops.

Some recent explanations of pain's chronicity utilize psychological concepts,[34] while others utilize neurophysiological concepts.[36] While the psychological explanations use concepts like fear-avoidance, catastrophizing, anxiety, and depression, the physiological explanations use concepts like allostasis and epigenetic changes, opioidergic and dopaminergic tone. But these different terms may mask an underlying similarity. Prognostic psychological concepts like catastrophizing have been associated with prognostic physiological concepts like central sensitization.[37] Catastrophizing adolescents show elevated fear and limbic activation in response to a learned threat cue. They also show decreased fronto-medial cortical activation and connectivity in response to a learned safety cue.[38] The ultimate similarity of physiological and psychological approaches may be especially important when it comes to treatment strategies. CBT has been shown to alter brain gray matter and improve functional connectivity in patients with chronic pain.[39,40] For this reason, Borsook and colleagues have asserted, "A closer partnership between behavioral and neurobiological science will benefit both."[36(p2425)]

These findings are consistent with the research reviewed above about pain perception utilizing the brain's salience network and being focused primarily on danger detection rather than damage detection. Tissue damage will often activate this danger detection system, but with wide variability in the amount of pain produced. Psychological variables like catastrophizing help explain this variability. Most acute injury does not result in chronic pain. Psychological models like fear avoidance and distress measures like anxiety and depression help explain the persistence of pain beyond healing time, as does a history of psychological trauma, especially childhood abuse.

Healing from physical trauma is relatively simple, and predictable enough that it is reasonable to assume that healing is complete 3 months after the trauma. This is the concept of "healing time" that Bonica used to distinguish acute from chronic pain. Healing from psychological trauma is not so simple or predictable. This is especially true if the trauma is repeated, occurs in childhood, or is perpetrated by trusted individuals. A broken leg has a more reliable and expected healing course than a broken heart. Recovery from childhood sexual abuse is prolonged and challenging because it requires re-establishing trust in relationships and trust in oneself.[41] Recovery from psychological trauma is difficult because the trauma is itself *morally* complex. A victim often also feels like a perpetrator. Victims may wonder if they invited or encouraged the abuse. Feelings about the trauma regularly include not only anger and sadness, but also guilt and shame. It is exceedingly difficult for these victims to feel safe again. In fact, after abuse, one's sense of safety and danger is so distorted that it is much more likely for women who were victims of childhood sexual abuse to be raped as adults.[42] This altered sense of safety and danger changes the victim's pain perception and pain behavior. It is common for child abuse victims to engage in non-suicidal self-injury, often self-cutting. Those who cut themselves explain that the physical pain produced by cutting is a welcome distraction from their ongoing psychic pain.

The strong evidence that psychological trauma increases the likelihood and severity of chronic pain is consistent with the view that chronic pain arises not from intra-body tissue damage, but rather from intrapersonal (i.e., homeostatic) *and* interpersonal danger. Danger and self-preservation are concepts that bridge the physiology–psychology divide. In a species as dependent on social support and cooperation as are humans, danger to bodily tissue includes physical and social threats. Indeed, it has been proposed that the human brain system that makes social rejection so painful for us likely exists as an evolutionary adaptation and extension of the physical pain mechanism found in simpler animals.[43] Physical pain and social pain serve to promote human survival, both as individuals and as a species.

If pain is a homeostatic emotion (concerning threats to bodily and personal integrity) like anxiety and depression, and they all share a common neurobiology, we understand them as a continuum of danger warnings, not as sensation and reaction. These homeostatic emotions have been honed through millions of years of natural selection to more efficiently support survival than any line-labeled system (pain vs. touch; nociceptive transmission vs. pain perception) that rigidly separates the processing of physical pain and social pain. As we have seen, pain can arise from physical or psychological trauma or both. Chronic pain remains a frustrating and intriguing clinical problem because it cannot be simply attributed to peripheral broken body parts or to centralized psychological states; often both are involved. Contrary to Descartes, clinical pain is continuously modulated by both the intrabody homeostatic environment and the interpersonal social environment. The endogenous opioid system is one of the principal means by which this modulation occurs. This is the main reason why opioids are such a potent pain treatment, and why they can be so harmful to full human functioning when used continuously and in the long term.

Suzanne Harris, part 6
___

Suzanne has less severe and frequent nightmares while taking prazosin, but her life remains very constricted. She continues to have abdominal pain and does not want to meet strangers or let anyone get close. She just doesn't feel safe. You suggest that psychotherapy for Suzanne's posttraumatic stress disorder is necessary for her to move beyond the physical and psychological trauma that she has suffered. She begins trauma-focused CBT, but she finds this difficult, and asks you why she must be dragged again through the trauma that she is trying to escape. It is bringing up all sorts of painful and complex feelings about her marriage and her miscarriage, in addition to awful images of the stabbing. You acknowledge that the therapy process is difficult, but it offers her the best chance of freeing herself from the emotional and physical pain of her trauma.

Reconciling impersonal and personal pain perception: danger and self-preservation

Proposing a biopsychosocial model of pain is not new nor is it new to invert it into a sociopsychobiological model, where social factors are more prominent.[44] But both of these models include only impersonal forces. (We reviewed the shortcomings of these models at the end of Chapter 5.) These models do not refer to personal intentions, identity, or interpersonal relationships. They therefore are expansions of the biomedical model, but do not overcome it to include an account of patients' personal experiences. To overcome the limits of the medical model and personalize the problem of chronic pain, we need to include personal as well as impersonal forces in our causal account of pain.

Truthfully, patients are asking for this. They ask not only "How do I have this pain?" but they also ask "Why do I have this pain?" For the clinician, this means including the choices, beliefs, and actions of the patient not as an afterthought or a supplement to mechanical pain models. Patients see these mechanical models as denials of the personal reality and significance of their pain. Psychology has followed physiology and physics in providing mechanical models of observed phenomena. Pain psychology research grants and journal articles often include diagrams of "psychological mechanisms" that are being studied. But patients don't see themselves or their values or choices in these diagrams. If we are to empower our patients to reclaim their lives from chronic pain, they need to be placed inside the model, not as spectators on the outside. We must find a way to answer both the "how" and the "why" of pain.

Wait! Isn't this turning the clock back to a prescientific model of pain as punishment? Doesn't this deepen rather than relieve the stigma suffered by patients with chronic pain? We have deployed the medical model of chronic pain, at least in part, to relieve suffering persons of responsibility, blame, and guilt for their condition. Similar efforts have been made to medicalize and destigmatize conditions like depression[45] and addiction.[46,47] We have moved these conditions out of the religious and moral domain to the medical domain precisely to reduce stigma and enhance care.

It is helpful to review studies of self-blame (stigma) and other-blame (injustice) to understand the social position of these patients and the moral dimension of their condition. In their recent review of the stigma associated with chronic pain, De Ruddere and Craig explain, "Stigmatizing responses are devaluing and discrediting responses of observers toward individuals who possess a particular characteristic that deviates from societal norms."[48(p1609)] In the case of chronic non-cancer pain, the relevant social norm is pain without a clear medical cause. The absence of a clear cause leads to doubt about this pain from healthcare professionals, relatives, friends, and even the patients themselves. This stigma is more than inconvenient or embarrassing because it is associated with underassessment and undertreatment of pain by clinicians.[49] Observers are especially likely to underestimate pain in patients who are considered responsible for their pain condtion.[50] These patients may be essentially rejected as legitimate patients and sent home to deal with their pain on their own.

Patients experiencing stigma with chronic pain are more likely to be depressed and more likely to be ashamed of being depressed.[51] Patients with chronic pain who feel stigmatized have lower self-esteem and pain self-efficacy. They are more likely to catastrophize about pain and report less personal control over pain. This is especially true in patients with chronic pain and depression,[52] who reported more negative beliefs about depression and depressed individuals as well as a desire to keep depression and their treatments secret from others. Patients with chronic pain and depression have great suffering, but are not validated by the medical model. Self-blame is of course one of the core symptoms of depression. Here we see it folding back on patients with chronic pain to further stigmatize and isolate them.

Blame for injury and chronic pain can also be directed outward toward others when there is a sense of injustice. Patients' perceptions of injustice concerning injury and chronic pain have been shown to be potent predictors of a wide variety of bad pain outcomes. Carriere and colleagues recently reviewed 34 studies of patients with work injury, whiplash injury, fibromyalgia, chronic musculoskeletal pain, osteoarthritis, and spinal cord injury.[53] These studies showed relationships between perceived injustice and pain severity, disability, and mental health problems. In some of these studies, these relationships were independent of established psychological factors like pain catastrophizing and fear of pain. A wide range of sources of injustice were found relevant, including the work supervisor, the driver of another vehicle, the health professional, the insurer, and family members.[54]

Injustice, like psychological trauma or abuse, can be understood as a form of social injury. Trust, fairness, or reciprocity is damaged and interpersonal relationships are disrupted. Here, suffering is experienced as unfair and undeserved. This social injury adds to physical injury to worsen and prolong pain and retard emotional and physical recovery. One way injustice appears to do this is by preventing pain acceptance. Indeed, in one study *all* of the effects of perceived injustice on physical function and opioid use were explained by the effect on pain acceptance.[55] Patients who feel their injury and pain are unjust have difficulty accepting their pain, resulting in more pain and more suffering. <u>Why</u> *this pain occurs thus shapes* <u>how</u> *it occurs.*

Suzanne Harris, part 7

Suzanne has been doing her trauma-focused therapy for a couple of months now. Her therapist has her focus on the worst parts of her stabbing: the fear she was going to be raped or killed or just sliced wide open. It has made her nightmares and panic attacks return. She pleads with you that neither the miscarriage nor the stabbing was her fault, so why must she go through this horrific treatment. Can't the pain just be taken away?

Blame for injury versus responsibility for recovery

Chronic pain is commonly accompanied by anxiety and depression, which is often interpreted as an understandable emotional reaction to a persistent aversive sensation. But this standard interpretation underestimates the kinship among these negative emotional states and leads us to misunderstand their social and moral dimensions. It portrays chronic pain as passive and innocent suffering produced by peripheral tissue damage. If anxiety and depression are interpreted as reasonable and understandable reactions to this pain, they can borrow some of the moral authority of chronic pain and be understood themselves as a form of innocent suffering.

More often anxiety and depression retain some taint of personal weakness or self-inflicted injury. Anxiety looks too much like cowardice and depression looks too much like laziness to be granted a free pass as innocent suffering. This moral dimension of mental illness has been thoughtfully discussed by anthropologist Tanya Luhrmann in her book on the tension between medical and psychodynamic models within American psychiatry, *Of Two Minds*.[56] She states: "We often find it difficult to respond to psychiatric patients as innocent sufferers because taking an overdose seems deliberate and chosen in a way that having cancer does not."[56(p271)] This is the reason patients with mental illness are often held more responsible for their suffering than patients with physical illness. This belief is remarkably persistent through history and widespread across cultures, even though many physical illnesses like lung cancer (from smoking) and diabetes (from obesity) have clear behavioral causes. To help us understand the differences in our moral interpretations of physical and mental illnesses, Luhrmann draws upon the distinction between inessential and essential suffering made by Martin Luther that we first mentioned in Chapters 1 and 2:

> Luther here used an old religious distinction, which I shall call the distinction between inessential and essential suffering, between the suffering that one can act on and suffering that, as a Catholic priest might say, one must offer up to God. Essential suffering is what we are not able to prevent but must survive if we can. Essential suffering is the inherent difficulty of human life ... Inessential suffering is the pain we can treat. ... Only suffering that is unavoidable must be accepted. ... As this distinction has been inherited by our Judeo-Christian culture, *medicine handles*

the inessential suffering, religion the essential suffering, and intentional
hurt falls into a limbo, neither treated by medicine nor tolerated by reli-
gion.[56(p272)] (emphasis added)

The medical model separates the source of the pain from the person and
treats it as inessential suffering. Within psychiatry, those who embrace the
medical model of depression treat it like a broken leg, something separate
from the person that can be repaired or expunged. This is a great gift, if
the source of the pain can be removed while leaving the person intact. But
if the depressive illness cannot be separated from the person, the promise
of the medical model is unfulfilled. Luhrmann explains, "The medical
model offers tremendous hope to those for whom a cure is found but con-
demns those whom a cure does not redeem.... We deprive them of their
sense of mastery over themselves, of full personhood in our world, of their
ability to see themselves as thinking and feeling, just differently from other
people."[56(p285)]

This hope and peril offered by the medical model to those with mental
illness apply to those with chronic pain as well. If the cause of the pain can
be removed, why not remove it? This hope supports not only back surgery
but opioid therapy for back pain. *That is why we call opioid analgesics "pain-*
killers." Patients demand painkillers because they want a medication that
takes away their pain but leaves them (as persons) alone. The problem is
that in the most common and difficult cases of chronic pain like nonspecific back pain and fibromyalgia, the cause can't be removed by surgery or
killed by opioids. Nor, as we have seen in the last chapter, do opioids leave
the person alone. The pain that the patient (and often the clinician) desperately wants to see as inessential suffering becomes over time more like
essential suffering, tied to their personhood. Paradoxically, this tie to personhood is especially true in those cases where it is argued that chronic pain
is not a symptom of disease, but has itself become a brain disease. This is
because there is no known means of removing the cause of this nociplastic or centralized pain without involving the person affected. Nociplastic
pain is thought to arise from a damaged or altered nociceptive system in
the brain. Although evidence of brain dysfunction in nociplastic pain syndromes like fibromyalgia has become much stronger in the past decade, we
have no drug or surgical therapies that reverse these processes. While antidepressant medications can be helpful, our best therapies for nociplastic

pain conditions are psychological and rehabilitative therapies that target the effects of these brain changes.

If chronic pain is essential suffering, "it is intrinsic to the person, to his experience of life, to his growth and future."[56(p252)] This makes the illness more morally complex, more individualized. But it does hold a benefit in "that the illness is not external, arbitrary, or other.... The illness, then, is not out of his control but something over which he is potentially a master." Since the illness is not an external imposition that can be removed without changing the person, it gives the person more ability to change the illness. Beliefs, behaviors, values, and habits all become relevant tools for recovery from chronic pain. Asserting that patients have a right to pain relief leaves them out of achieving that pain relief. This right to pain relief denies that patient agency is relevant to recovery. The patient with a chronic illness cannot succeed as the passive recipient of a medical cure, but must participate in the recovery process.

The value of this participation is not limited to mental illnesses.[57] Participation is valuable in many chronic illnesses, such as diabetes, where it is not possible for the clinicians to simply "fix" the patient. This is also true of depressive patients, who are encouraged to change comforting but self-defeating avoidance behaviors, and protective but self-defeating beliefs, and counterproductive sleep habits. All of these changes are also relevant to chronic pain care. A passive diabetic patient who takes his pills but does nothing to change his diet and exercise habits will be unlikely to do well. A hypertensive patient who takes medication but remains sedentary and obese is less likely to lower his blood pressure. In these chronic illnesses, as in chronic pain, many factors beyond the patient's control, including genetics, intrauterine environment, early family support, neighborhood resources, and economic opportunities, may help cause trauma and pain. Patients are not responsible for these, but patients are accountable for participation in their recovery.

What is likely to be most effective for patients is a *forward-looking* responsibility rather than a *backward-looking* blaming. This model of "responsibility without blame" has been developed by philosopher Hanna Pickard.[58] She argues that this model of forward-looking care applies especially to "disorders of agency" (personality disorders, addiction, eating disorders). "Core diagnostic symptoms of maintaining factors of disorders of agency are actions and omissions: patterns of behavior central to the nature or maintenance of the condition."[58(p1134)] But any chronic illness, physical or mental, involves patient agency. All chronic illnesses require patient agency to be part of the healing process.[57]

With these *morally complex* chronic illnesses, "clinicians can often find themselves trapped between a *desire to rescue* and a *desire to blame*, despite neither response being clinically effective."[58(p1142)] The desire to rescue (typical of the medical model) arises from an underestimation of patient agency concerning the illness that absolves the patient of any responsibility for recovery. This desire to rescue is what motivates clinicians to write opioid prescriptions for chronic pain.[59] Clinicians can try so hard to avoid blaming patients that they exclude the patient from the recovery process. Clinicians and patients alike love to find something on the MRI scan that is causing the pain, not only because it raises the possibility of cure, but also because the lesion is exculpatory for the patient. It proves her pain is real and not her fault.

Clinicians must hold patients accountable for their recovery without blaming them for their illness. This balance is also essential for successful care of addicted patients and includes "an attitude of calm respect, that helps them both think and talk with [patients] about their responsibility for harmful behavior, without blaming them."[58(p1150)] Compassion and empathy are effective antidotes to blaming. They are achieved by listening to and understanding the patient's story, including stories of both physical and psychological trauma and any accompanying protective homeostatic emotions like anxiety and depression. *The focus is not upon validating pain by tying it to an adequate physical cause (as per above discussions of pain stigma), but in validating and addressing the sources of danger in the patient's life: "What is making you feel unsafe as a body and a person these days?"*

This kind of accountability can be empowering for patients *if they see it as a way to reclaim their distinctive life*. We have found this in our treatment trial of our online PainTracker Self-Manager.[60] One step in this pain self-management support intervention is a values clarification exercise. In this exercise, patients are encouraged to step out of the survival-focused "perpetual crisis" into which many patients with complex chronic pain may slip. In this crisis mode, they set aside the values and passions that define them as a person to focus on simply surviving from day to day. They forget who they are as distinctive individuals as they simply try to survive from Monday to Tuesday. In our values clarification exercise, they are encouraged to step out of crisis mode by reclaiming the values and passions that define them as a person. This reactivation of their identity and values helps make resuming life, even including pain, more desirable and possible. "One lesson that clearly can be learned from clinical contexts is this: we do not help [patients] with disorders of agency by denying their agency and absolving them from responsibility."[58(p1148)] Our treatment models must make room for the agency that we are trying to foster.[57] Telling patients that they have a brain disease called chronic pain or ICD-11 Chronic Primary Pain may or may not destigmatize their condition, but it does not empower them by clarifying the role that they can play in their own recovery. It may in fact instill fatalism and passivity since it is not clear to patients how changing their beliefs and behavior can cure a brain disease.

Opioid therapy as the answer to the innocent suffering of chronic pain

During the first decade of the 21st century, primary care clinicians often encountered patients with chronic pain seeking care who asked difficult and provocative questions: *Do you not believe I am in pain? Do you not believe that I deserve relief?* Many clinicians at that time felt that it was not possible to answer "no" to either of these questions, so they felt unable to refuse patients' requests for opioid therapy. By the year 2000, it was no longer legitimate to doubt a patient's pain simply because a causal lesion could not be found on the MRI scan. And it was not allowed to deny a *living* patient's request for legitimate pain relief, since it was not allowed to deny a *dying* patient's legitimate claim for palliative pain relief. Purdue Pharma marketing material referred frequently to "legitimate pain patients" and their rightful quest for "legitimate pain relief." We have hopefully clarified some of the complex issues and assumptions that lie behind these deceptively simple patient questions. We have hopefully clarified the righteousness of the claim to a right to pain relief. Even the modern effort to provide pain relief based on impersonal pain mechanisms is haunted by questions concerning personal responsibility for suffering.

We are certainly not advocating that clinicians start with doubt about patients' pain complaints. In established outpatient practice, malingering is very rare. We are strongly arguing against the idea that patients' pain can or should be validated through correspondence with tissue damage. Assessing the "reality" of the patient's pain is not the central challenge of chronic pain care. Validating pain through functional MRI scans of patients' brains is as big a mistake as validating back pain through structural MRI scans of patients' spines. Assessing the "reality" of a patient's depression is similarly not the central challenge of depression care. The central challenge is finding a way for the patient to move his life forward. This may seem nebulous because moving life forward can take many forms: returning to work, having fun, making friends, volunteering, finding new or old hobbies. Increasing the patient's capacity for personally meaningful action reduces pain salience and often pain intensity.[61]

Asserting a patient's right to pain relief is complex. Palliative care advocates convinced the American public, and the Supreme Court, that *dying in great pain* is a grievous moral harm and government has an obligation to reduce this pain. Opioid therapy can help provide this relief. These same advocates then convinced us that *living in great pain* is also a grievous moral harm. Opioid therapy was to rectify this harm as well. We saw this painful living as a medical problem that demanded a medical solution. What is wrong with this extension of the right of pain relief?

The error concerns the nature of recovery from chronic pain. This recovery requires patient participation. Passive submission to professional care is not adequate. Perhaps it is adequate in acute illnesses like pneumonia, but not in chronic illnesses like diabetes. This passive submission seems reasonable only when we understand chronic pain as a form of innocent suffering, separable from the rest of human suffering, about which the patient can do nothing on his own. This physical pain arises from impersonal mechanical forces over which the patient has no control. He therefore presents himself for medical care where he may claim a right to pain relief. We hear this claim much more often than a claim to a right to anxiety relief or a right to depression relief. This is because patient participation in recovery is thought more important for these undeniably personal "mental" disorders. We don't hear of rights to relief of suffering or rights to relief of stress because we recognize these as inescapable components of human life that have many non-medical causes and remedies. *Not all human suffering can be addressed medically.*

A claim to a right to pain relief is also more likely because we grant a strange moral privilege to *localized* suffering. If it hurts in a specific place on your body, you have a more valid claim to medical relief than if the pain cannot be localized. Before they dispense opioids, clinicians want to know (as did Pink Floyd): *Can you show me where it hurts?* Because of the kinship of localized pain with that of acute injury, it is thought to be independent of the person. Since around 1800, medical science has looked to tissue damage as revealed by the autopsy or one of its modern imaging surrogates as the definitive evidence of disease and the cause for its symptoms.[62] Beginning in the 19th century, those persons with symptoms or suffering, but without identifiable disease, were triaged away from the scientific hospital and its clinics. In the 21st century, chronic pain care still dwells in this regime of objective disease, even though we have learned that objective tissue damage is neither a necessary nor sufficient cause for chronic pain. If we are constrained by these 19th-century options to designate chronic pain as either a symptom of disease or as a disease in itself, it makes sense to choose the latter.[63] But this dichotomy predates all the modern pain research that undercuts it. Chronic pain is neither disease nor symptom but a condition or illness. It need not be forced onto the side of objective disease or onto the side of subjective symptom.

The way to bring the person back into chronic pain care is not to remoralize the pain experience. We do not want to return to the idea of pain as punishment for sins, either personal or original. But we do want to make space for patients to ask: "What can I do and what should I do?" If patients are not asking these questions, we want to help them understand how important they are to their recovery. Occasionally chronic pain can be cured through a procedure or a medication, but this is unusual and should not distort the entire enterprise of chronic pain care. Some chronic low back pain can be cured through spine surgery, but the vast majority cannot.[63]

Fibromyalgia is best understood as a chronic illness.[64] It does not help to force it into the physical illness or mental illness categories. Like other chronic illnesses such as diabetes, fibromyalgia treatment must encompass the patient's lifestyle, behavior, even identity. Fibromyalgia cannot be cured by a procedure despite being the prototypical nociplastic, centralized, "chronic pain as itself a disease" state. In our clinical experience, both sleep and exercise are crucial to recovery from fibromyalgia. Some prescribed medications (antidepressants, but not opioids or benzodiazepines) may be helpful in improving sleep, but these are rarely enough unless activity tolerance also increases through exercise.[65] Physicians may prescribe the pills, but the patients need to exercise. Patient participation in recovery is essential.[66]

Opioids decrease patient participation in rehabilitation. In the 1990s, many of us believed that initial opioid treatment of injured workers would promote rehabilitation and return to work by providing pain relief and enabling participation in physical therapy. Unfortunately, this is not true. At least seven prospective cohort studies have shown that early opioid prescription retards rather than promotes return to work among injured workers.[67] This is because the deactivating effect of opioids may be greater than the analgesic effect. This is another reason why interpreting a right to pain relief as a right to opioid therapy is mistaken. Although opioids have been nicknamed "painkillers," they don't kill pain and leave the person intact. They have widespread effects throughout the human nervous and endocrine system, inhibiting some of our most distinctive human functions that are dependent on the endogenous opioid system such as social bonding, empathy, and emotion discrimination.[68] Opioids, when used long term, may be "brainkillers" more than painkillers.

Suzanne Harris, part 8

Six months after her last visit Suzanne returns, looking animated and lively. She says her trauma-focused therapy is continuing, but she and her therapist have finished talking about the stabbing. The therapy is now focused on her choice of a husband who hit her sometimes and her sometimes violent father. As she worked through her trauma, the pervasive sense of threat and danger that had dominated her life began to fade. And her abdominal pain, though it didn't disappear, became less of a barrier to her life, which now includes some new friends she met through yoga.

Conclusion: reintegrating chronic pain with the rest of human suffering

Our modern approach to pain has been a medical approach, rooted in biological explanations concerning mechanical processes within the body. This focus on medical diagnoses and physiological causes has been supplemented by reference to psychological factors and social influences in what has become known as the biopsychosocial model of pain. But biological, psychological, and social causes are not treated equally in this model. Biological, intrabody causes are given priority over psychological and social interpersonal causes. And in many primary care settings, which is where most chronic pain care is delivered, the biomedical approach to chronic pain is still dominant. This means that we have left the person out of our explanations for chronic pain. As modern scientists, we answer questions about "how" someone came to have chronic pain, but ignore questions about "why" someone came to have chronic pain. We are more comfortable with questions about mechanisms than questions about meanings. We have set up chronic pain as a form of innocent suffering for which the prescription of opioid painkillers makes moral sense.

Chronic pain is a morally complex condition. It is not childhood cancer. On the other hand, it is not pedophilia. It is like diabetes or depression or a thousand other chronic illnesses that can rarely be cured. These conditions are caused by genetics and many other factors over which patients have no control. But recovery does depend on patient agency and participation. Without personal attention to beliefs and behaviors and lifestyle, recovery may be stymied. An effort to kill this pain with opioids—in accord with a right to pain relief—may undermine the initiative and social function that are the paths back to a productive and satisfying life.

Pain is a nearly universal human experience, tied to our vulnerability to death and disease. We have made great strides over the last century in understanding how tissue damage is encoded in nociception and transmitted to the CNS. We understand some aspects of the process by which nociception becomes pain perception. But we have not been able to find pain-specific structures and processes in the brain. Pain perception becomes intertwined with other forms of danger perception in a salience network that encodes any sensory information that is relevant to our survival. Pain and other suffering are unified as homeostatic emotions that signal when our biological, personal, or social integrity is threatened. Our efforts to reduce pain and suffering are most likely to succeed when we address the intrabody and interpersonal roots of human suffering as a unified whole.

References

1. Wall P. *Pain: The Science of Suffering.* Columbia University Press; 2002.
2. Casey KL. *Chasing Pain: The Search for a Neurobiological Mechanism.* Oxford University Press; 2019.
3. Melzack R, Wall PD. Pain mechanisms: a new theory. *Science.* 1965;150:971–979.
4. Basbaum A. Specificity versus patterning theory: continuing the debate. *Pain Research Forum.* 2011. https://www.painresearchforum.org/forums/discussion/7347-specificity-versus-patterning-theory-continuing-debate
5. Noe A. *Action in Perception.* MIT Press; 2004.
6. Aydede M. What is a pain in a body part? *Can J Philos.* 2020;50(2):143–158.
7. Ramachandran VS, Blakeslee S. *Phantoms in the Brain: Probing the Mysteries of the Human Mind.* William Morrow; 1998.
8. Dennett DC. *Consciousness Explained.* Little Brown; 1991.
9. Fuchs T. *Ecology of the Brain.* Oxford University Press; 2018.
10. Kucyi A, Davis KD. The neural code for pain: from single-cell electrophysiology to the dynamic pain connectome. *Neuroscientist.* 2017;23(4):397–414.
11. Borsook D, Edwards R, Elman I, et al. Pain and analgesia: the value of salience circuits. *Prog Neurobiol.* 2013;104:93–105.
12. Legrain V, Iannetti GD, Plaghki L, Mouraux A. The pain matrix reloaded: a salience detection system for the body. *Prog Neurobiol.* 2011;93:111–124.
13. Iannetti GD, Mouraux A. From the neuromatrix to the pain matrix (and back). *Exp Brain Res.* 2010;205:1–12.
14. Hubbard CS, Lazaridou A, Cahalan CM, et al. Aberrant salience? Brain hyperactivation in response to pain onset and offset in fibromyalgia. *Arthritis Rheumatol.* 2020;72:1203–1213.
15. Menon V. Salience network. In: Toga AW, ed. *Brain Mapping: An Encyclopedic Reference.* Vol. 2. Academic Press, Elsevier; 2015:597–611.
16. Cohen M, Quintner J, Buchanan D. Is chronic pain a disease? *Pain Med.* 2013;14:1284–1288.
17. Butler DS, Moseley L. *Explain Pain.* Noigroup Publications; 2013.
18. Moseley GL, Butler DS. Fifteen years of explaining pain: the past, present, and future. *J Pain.* 2015;16:807–813.
19. Lee H, McAuley J, Hübscher M, et al. Does changing pain-related knowledge reduce pain and improve function through changes in catastrophizing? *Pain.* 2016;157:922–930.

20. Moseley GL, Nicholas MK, Hodges PW. A randomized controlled trial of intensive neurophysiology education in chronic low back pain. *Clin J Pain.* 2004;20:324–330.

21. Louw A, Diener I, Butler DS, Puentedura EJ. The effect of neuroscience education on pain, disability, anxiety, and stress in chronic musculoskeletal pain. *Arch Phys Med Rehabil.* 2011;92:2041–2056.

22. Baliki MN, Apkarian AV. Nociception, pain, negative moods, and behavior selection. *Neuron.* 2015;87:474–491.

23. Coenen VA, Schlaepfer TE, Maedler B, Panksepp J. Cross-species affective functions of the medial forebrain bundle: implications for the treatment of affective pain and depression in humans. *Neurosci Biobehav Rev.* 2011;35:1971–1981.

24. Craig AD. How do you feel? Interoception: the sense of the physiological condition of the body. *Nature Rev Neurosci.* 2002;3:655–666.

25. Porreca F, Navratilova E. Reward, motivation, and emotion of pain and its relief. *Pain.* 2017;158(Suppl 1):S43–S49.

26. Melzack R, Casey KL. Sensory, motivational, and central control determinant of pain: a new conceptual model. In: Kenshalo DR, ed. *Skin Senses: Proceedings of the First International Symposium on the Skin Senses.* Charles C. Thomas; 1968:423–439.

27. Klein C. *What the Body Commands: The Imperative Theory of Pain.* MIT Press; 2015.

28. Barwich AS. *Smellosophy: What the Nose Tells the Mind.* Harvard University Press; 2020.

29. Ballantyne JC, Sullivan MD. The discovery of endogenous opioid systems: what it has meant for understanding pain and its treatment. *Pain.* 2017;158(12):2290–2300.

30. Bonica J. *The Management of Pain.* Lea and Febiger; 1953.

31. Heitmann H, May ES, Tiemann L, et al. Motor responses to noxious stimuli shape pain perception in chronic pain patients. *eNeuro.* 2018;5(5):eneuro.0290-18.2018.

32. Walters ET, Williams ACC. Evolution of mechanisms and behaviour important for pain. *Philos Trans R Soc Lond B Biol Sci.* 2019;374:20190275.

33. Fillingim RB. Individual differences in pain: understanding the mosaic that makes pain personal. *Pain.* 2017;158(Suppl 1):S11–S18.

34. Edwards RR, Dworkin RH, Sullivan MD, et al. The role of psychosocial processes in the development and maintenance of chronic pain. *J Pain.* 2016;17:T70–T92.

35. Adler-Neal AL, Emerson NM, Farris SR, et al. Brain moderators supporting the relationship between depressive mood and pain. *Pain.* 2019;160:2028–2035.

36. Borsook D, Youssef AM, Simons L, et al. When pain gets stuck: the evolution of pain chronification and treatment resistance. *Pain.* 2018;159:2421–2436.

37. Meints SM, Mawla I, Napadow V, et al. The relationship between catastrophizing and altered pain sensitivity in patients with chronic low-back pain. *Pain.* 2019;160:833–843.

38. Heathcote LC, Timmers I, Kronman CA, et al. Brain signatures of threat-safety discrimination in adolescent chronic pain. *Pain.* 2020;161:630–640.

39. Seminowicz DA, Shpaner M, Keaser ML, et al. Cognitive-behavioral therapy increases prefrontal cortex gray matter in patients with chronic pain. *J Pain.* 2013;14:1573–1584.

40. Shpaner M, Kelly C, Lieberman G, et al. Unlearning chronic pain: a randomized controlled trial to investigate changes in intrinsic brain connectivity following cognitive behavioral therapy. *Neuroimage Clin.* 2014;5:365–376.

41. Arias BJ, Johnson CV. Voices of healing and recovery from childhood sexual abuse. *J Child Sex Abuse.* 2013;22:822–841.

42. Coid J, Petruckevitch A, Feder G, et al. Relation between childhood sexual and physical abuse and risk of revictimisation in women: a cross-sectional survey. *Lancet.* 2001;358:450–454.

43. Eisenberger NI. The pain of social disconnection: examining the shared neural underpinnings of physical and social pain. *Nat Rev Neurosci.* 2012;13:421–434.

44. Carr DB, Bradshaw YS. Time to flip the pain curriculum? *Anesthesiology.* 2014;120:12–14.

45. Mann SL, Contrada RJ. Biological causal beliefs and depression stigma: the moderating effects of first- and second-hand experience with depression. *J Ment Health.* 2022;31(1):5–13.

46. Kreek MJ, Reed B, Butelman ER. Current status of opioid addiction treatment and related preclinical research. *Sci Adv.* 2019;5:eaax9140.

47. Frank LE, Nagel SK. Addiction and moralization: the role of the underlying model of addiction. *Neuroethics.* 2017;10:129–139.

48. De Ruddere L, Craig KD. Understanding stigma and chronic pain: a-state-of-the-art review. *Pain.* 2016;157:1607–1610.

49. De Ruddere L, Goubert L, Stevens MA, et al. Health care professionals' reactions to patient pain: impact of knowledge about medical evidence and psychosocial influences. *J Pain.* 2014;15:262–270.

50. De Ruddere L, Goubert L, Stevens M, et al. Discounting pain in the absence of medical evidence is explained by negative evaluation of the patient. *Pain.* 2013;154:669–676.

51. Waugh OC, Byrne DG, Nicholas MK. Internalized stigma in people living with chronic pain. *J Pain.* 2014;15:550 e1–e10.

52. Naushad N, Dunn LB, Munoz RF, Leykin Y. Depression increases subjective stigma of chronic pain. *J Affect Disord.* 2018;229:456–462.

53. Carriere JS, Donayre Pimentel S, Yakobov E, Edwards RR. A systematic review of the association between perceived injustice and pain-related outcomes in individuals with musculoskeletal pain. *Pain Med.* 2020;21:1449–1463.

54. Sullivan MJL. Perceptions of injustice and problematic pain outcomes. *Pain Med.* 2020;21:1315–1336.

55. Carriere JS, Sturgeon JA, Yakobov E, et al. The impact of perceived injustice on pain-related outcomes: A combined model examining the mediating roles of pain acceptance and anger in a chronic pain sample. *Clin J Pain.* 2018;34:739–747.

56. Luhrmann TM. *Of Two Minds: The Growing Disorder in American Psychiatry.* Alfred A. Knopf; 2000.

57. Sullivan MD. *Patient as Agent of Health and Health Care.* Oxford University Press; 2017.

58. Pickard H. Responsibility without blame: philosophical reflections on clinical practice In: Fulford K, ed. *Oxford Handbook of Philosophy and Psychiatry.* Oxford University Press; 2013:1134–1152.

59. Hooten WM, Brummett CM, Sullivan MD, et al. A conceptual framework for understanding unintended prolonged opioid use. *Mayo Clin Proc.* 2017;92:1822–1830.

60. Sullivan M, Langford DJ, Davies PS, et al. A controlled pilot trial of PainTracker Self-Manager, a web-based platform combined with patient coaching, to support patients' self-management of chronic pain. *J Pain.* 2018;19:996–1005.

61. Sullivan MD, Vowles KE. Patient action: as means and end for chronic pain care. *Pain.* 2017;158:1405–1407.

62. Foucault M. *The Birth of the Clinic: An Archaeology of Medical Perception.* Vintage Books; 1973.

63. Clauw DJ, Essex MN, Pitman V, Jones KD. Reframing chronic pain as a disease, not a symptom: rationale and implications for pain management. *Postgrad Med.* 2019;131:185–198.

64. Clauw DJ, D'Arcy Y, Gebke K, et al. Normalizing fibromyalgia as a chronic illness. *Postgrad Med.* 2018;130:9–18.

65. Clauw DJ. Fibromyalgia: a clinical review. *JAMA.* 2014;311:1547–1555.

66. Vader K, Patel R, Doulas T, Miller J. Promoting participation in physical activity and exercise among people living with chronic pain: A qualitative study of strategies used by people with pain and their recommendations for health care providers. *Pain Med.* 2020;21:625–635.

67. Franklin GM, Fulton-Kehoe D, Turner JA, Wickizer T. Prescription opioid use and the risk of disability. *Clin J Pain.* 2018;34:190.

68. Sullivan MD, Ballantyne JC. When physical and social pain coexist: insights into opioid therapy. *Ann Fam Med.* 2021;19(1):79–82.

9
Finding a place for pain in medicine, in policy, and in life

> But what if pleasure and pain should be so closely connected that he who wants the greatest possible amount of the one must also have the greatest possible amount of the other, that he who wants to experience the "heavenly high jubilation," must also be ready to be "sorrowful unto death"?
>
> Friedrich Nietzsche, *The Gay Science* (Figure 9.1)

Introduction: finding a place for pain

Someday there'll be a cure for pain
That's the day I throw my drugs away
When they find a cure for pain

Cure for Pain, by Morphine

We hope for a cure for pain, specifically a cure for chronic pain. That is what our patients hope for. They tell us that they would have no interest in opioids if we could just find the cause for their pain and remove it. This reveals that opioids are functioning as a substitute for a chronic pain cure. Indeed, we medicalize pain in order to remove it. Medicalization includes the implicit promise of removal. We separate pain as a mechanical medical phenomenon from the person so we can remove or kill the pain and leave the person alone.

Is all pain bad? The utilitarians thought so. Those who advocated for pain as a fifth vital sign in medical settings also implied that pain should always be reduced to a minimum. Many pain medicine physicians argue that acute pain serves a useful protective function, but that chronic pain provides benefit to no one and so should be eliminated or minimized. Before the secularism of

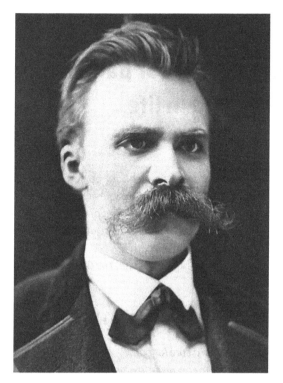

Figure 9.1. Friedrich Nietzsche
https://commons.wikimedia.org/wiki/File:Nietzsche187a.jpg. Friedrich Hermann
Hartmann, Public domain, via Wikimedia Commons

modern society became dominant, the Catholic Church taught us that pain
cleansed our souls of sin and prepared the way for our eternal salvation. Now
we are told that pain relief is among the core universal human rights that
should be provided by all societies.

This raises the question: Where should pain fit into a good human life?
Americans believe that allowing patients to die in severe, uncontrolled pain
is morally unacceptable. The Supreme Court has agreed. American doctors were convinced by opioid advocates from the palliative care world that
allowing patients to live in severe uncontrolled pain was also morally unacceptable. But deploying opioids to relieve this chronic pain has not significantly reduced the population's burden of pain and has increased its burden

of misery through overdose, addiction, and social impairments related to opioid dependence. Were health professionals just mistaken that opioids were a safe and effective treatment for chronic pain or did they make a bigger mistake about the place of pain in a good human life? The argument of this book is that health professionals have misunderstood not only opioids, but also pain itself.

Daniel Perkins, part 1

Daniel is a 48-year-old male, newly moved to Seattle. He reports back, neck, and head pain since a motor vehicle accident 8 years ago. His spinal magnetic resonance imaging (MRI) scans show degenerative changes, but nothing that can be surgically repaired. He reports 10/10 pain, which he states has produced moderately severe depression and hopelessness. He tells you that physical therapy and antidepressant medications have not worked. He did have trouble with alcohol, but that was before the accident. He has now been sober for 10 years. He asks to continue the oxycodone ER 40 mg twice daily prescribed by his doctor in Tulsa, which he says helps. He says he has never lost a prescription or asked for an early refill and invites you to confirm this with his Tulsa doctor. He senses your hesitation and challenges you: Don't you believe I am in pain? Don't you believe that I deserve relief?

If you were Daniel's doctor, what do you owe to Daniel? Do you owe him a cure? This would be wonderful and satisfying to everyone, but is possible only in a small percentage of chronic pain cases. Do you owe him a diagnosis? This also would be welcome and satisfying. But many chronic pain diagnoses are either irrelevant (bulging disc) or vague (myofascial pain) or invalid (lumbar sprain). These diagnoses often don't help identify effective treatments or provide a reliable prognosis. Perhaps if neither a cure nor a diagnosis is available, we can at least provide pain relief. But how much pain relief is needed and at what cost? For pain relief always has a cost. If we lower pain levels, and also lower functional capacity through sedation and passivity, has the patient gained anything?

Maybe we should follow the International Association for the Study of Pain's Declaration of Montreal and promise not painkilling or even pain relief, but only pain management. Then we must ask: What tools will be used, with what goals? Pain management can mean anything or nothing, and it is rarely something patients ask for. Patients want their pain relieved, not managed. Some experts suggest that we look beyond the pain experience and instead offer Daniel improved function. But we must ask again: What kind of function, aimed at which goals? In chronic pain care, "function" is often shorthand for physical function, meaning the ability to move and possibly work. However, meaningful human function also includes cognitive, emotional, and social function. These are also impaired in many cases of complex chronic pain, but can be further impaired by opioid treatment of that pain. Maybe we should aim for something broader, like a better quality of life for Daniel. This is more personally meaningful, yet we must ask: Quality of life as defined by whom and according to what standard?

In any thoughtful reconsideration of the goals of chronic pain clinical care, we are pushed outward from our traditional focus on damage, nociception, and pain to consider the context within which these occur. This contextualization of chronic pain *goals* parallels the contextualization of chronic pain *mechanisms* that we reviewed in Chapter 8. Pain care, pain science, and pain policy all must reach beyond the boundaries of the human body to consider pain's role in human life. In Chapter 8, we found that we could only understand the variable relationship between pain and damage if we understood how it related to the survival of the organism and the species. In this chapter, we will also find that the answer to technical problems in pain care require a deeper understanding of the human context within which they arise. We will work our way backward through the Western history of pain, gradually unwinding the tight knots of pain problems bequeathed to us: from pain conceived as a medical problem, to pain as a social problem, and finally to pain as an existential or religious problem.

Unwinding the right to the reduction of quantified medical pain

I was plunged into degrees of pain and realistic depression that produced a dangerously passive state. In that psychic bog of helplessness, like most trapped sufferers, I was transfixed by the main sight in view—my undiminished physical pain. And in such a trance state, for that's what a heavily drugged life is, any personal crusade for sane alternative therapies was literally unthinkable to me. It was all I could do to focus my scarce strength and clarity on one main aim beyond plain endurance, pain relief.

Reynolds Price, *A Whole New Life*

Reynolds Price (Figure 9.2) was a Duke University English professor and prize-winning novelist who developed severe neuropathic pain after he had a spinal tumor resected and radiated. As he describes eloquently above, his

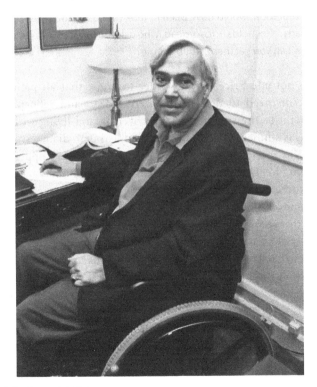

Figure 9.2. Reynolds Price

rich life shrunk down to the single-minded pursuit of pain relief. This capacity of pain to shrink life down to the pursuit of pain reduction is why the right to pain relief has moral power. How can any life be possible for someone like Price without pain relief? The remainder of his book describes how he was prescribed many different medications (including opioids) and received many non-pharmacological treatments like hypnosis and cognitive–behavioral therapy for the treatment of his chronic pain. The medications (opioids, benzodiazepines, amitriptyline, among others) provided some pain relief, but at the cost of sedation and mental dulling that he found unacceptable.

Ultimately, he discovered that he needed to change his therapeutic goal of reducing pain. He learned that something more radical was necessary. He needed to completely reinvent himself:

> The kindest thing anyone could have done for me, once I'd finished five weeks' radiation, would have been to look me square in the eye and say this clearly, "Reynolds Price is dead. Who will you be now? Who *can* you be and how can you get there, double-time?"[1(p126)]

We do not cite Price here in order to argue that all patients with chronic pain need to declare themselves dead and reborn. We cite him to point to the complexity of recovering and living with chronic pain. This is similar to the challenge of adjusting to diabetes. Instead of asking "Why me?", he learned to ask "What next?" He stopped fighting and denying his paraplegia and his pain and found a way back into his writing work.

Sometimes chronic pain can be cured, but more often it cannot. It is often a process that requires reaching inside oneself to change not just beliefs and behaviors, but even one's identity. We have oversimplified chronic pain by depersonalizing its assessment and treatment. This implies that we can reduce or eliminate chronic pain without changing the person with the pain. The great promise of the biomedical model as applied to chronic pain is that this pain is inessential suffering that can be safely and expeditiously eliminated. It promises that chronic pain can be killed with pills or procedures while leaving the person untouched. This promise is one of the deep roots of our opioid epidemic.

Abandon clinical outpatient use of pain intensity scores

The 0-to-10 pain intensity scale that has become a familiar feature of clinical care had its origin in experimental psychophysics studies that investigated the relationship between noxious stimulus intensity and pain experience. In acute postoperative care, this scale may have improved pain control in the days immediately following surgery. In palliative care and cancer pain care, the scale was combined with the "titrate to effect" opioid dosing principle to aggressively target pain levels in seriously ill patients with poor prognoses. It began to seriously distort clinical pain care only when it was extended to the outpatient care of patients with chronic non-cancer pain. Cancer pain treatment in the 1980s was simpler due to its clear origin in progressive tissue destruction and short time frame of treatment at the end of life. We have discussed above how this 0-to-10 pain intensity metric neglects important aspects of pain (e.g., meaning, extent, constancy), isolates pain and its treatment from their effect on the patient's life, and selects high-risk patients for the riskiest opioid regimens.[2] Although these scores have been repeatedly shown not to improve chronic pain care as was hoped, they continue to be used in most healthcare systems. We believe these scores should be phased out in favor of more personalized and qualitative measures, applied only when pain is the focus of clinical care.

Use of a simple quantitative pain metric, such as the pain intensity score, makes clinical pain assessment simple and allows averaging across populations of patients. It makes certain clinical epidemiology and quality improvement projects possible. But it also distorts these projects because it implies that zero pain is the goal. Or the scale is combined with policy that sets another arbitrary threshold for pain requiring clinical attention (such as 4/10 that the Veterans Administration used in the past). All these score-focused strategies err by isolating the goals of chronic pain care from the patient's life.

One of the briefest alternatives to the 0-to-10 pain intensity score is the 3-item PEG scale, adapted from the longer Brief Pain Inventory (BPI) used in many clinical pain research studies. It has been shown to capture almost all the information of the longer BPI when used in a primary care setting.[3] This scale adds two more 0-to-10 scales to a 0-to-10 "Pain severity" scale. One asks how much the pain interferes with "Enjoyment of life," the other with "General activities." The total PEG score thus provides a fuller picture of the effect of pain on the patient's life by adding assessments of role function and emotional function. It begins to refocus care away from the sensation of pain and onto the patient with pain. While the PEG is an important improvement on the pain intensity scale, hopefully we will see more feasible comprehensive personalized pain measures developed.

More broadly, we must ask if it makes sense, or advances the goal of pain relief, to measure pain when the clinical context is not one where pain is expected. This has become common as part of the effort to increase the "visibility" of pain in clinical settings. But does it make sense to ask the patient presenting for a routine eye exam or flu shot "Do you have any pain?" This assumes that all pain is a medical problem with a medical solution. During most routine visits, there is not time to delve into the context of the patient's pain or even treat the pain appropriately—at best, a note to the patient's primary care provider, if there is one, or perhaps a referral to a pain clinic, if there is one. Maybe the only thing these universally required pain questions have done is reinforce the contemporary belief that we shouldn't have any pain, and if we do, it should have a medical solution.

Redefine the medical necessity of pain treatment

If pain treatment is not mandated by a pain intensity score, what should indicate the need for pain treatment, especially opioid treatment? The Joint Commission, which accredits hospitals and other healthcare institutions, has begun to grapple with this issue. In 2001, the Joint Commission infamously recommended the use of quantitative pain scales to monitor patients' pain in hospitals.[4] Their recommendation contributed to the widespread use of the 0-to-10 pain intensity scale in hospitals and clinics. The new standards proposed in 2018 specifically recommend pain assessment and treatment standards tied to functional outcomes.[5] In the hospital, patients' pain should be controlled not to zero or some other arbitrarily defined minimum, but to promote relevant functions such as breathing, coughing, weight bearing, and walking. These criteria help determine when patients can be discharged from the hospital to home, so they are the appropriate criteria for pain management in the hospital.

The medical necessity of pain treatment outside the hospital is more complicated because life outside the hospital is more complicated. At a minimum, we must distinguish between common chronic pain and high-impact chronic pain, which only includes pain with daily functional limitations. While chronic pain itself has a prevalence of 20% in the United States, high-impact chronic pain has a prevalence of 8%.[6] This high-impact group with significant functional limitations has more need for medical treatment than those with chronic pain alone. Nevertheless, in every case, the functional gain achieved through pain treatment must be weighed against any short-term or long-term functional deficits produced through the pain treatment. When considering opioids, these deficits can include immediately apparent and obvious effects like sedation and less immediately obvious effects like opioid dependence or social and emotional impairments.

The medical necessity of pain treatment needs to be determined by the effects of the pain, not by its intensity or its causes. This conflicts with the usual way we demarcate medical problems from non-medical problems in our society. Classically, medical problems consist of diseases or injuries causing symptoms. But a causal disease often cannot be identified for chronic pain. So we can't understand the medical necessity of pain treatment if we stay locked into the disease-versus-symptom thinking typical of the biomedical model. Chronic pain is neither a disease nor just the symptom of another disease. That is what makes it complicated. To move forward with chronic pain care, we must break out of the "pain as symptom or disease" dichotomy. As Bill Fordyce used to say, chronic pain is "transdermal." It has causes inside the body and outside the body. Fordyce also taught us that treating the functional impairments produced by pain is one way to treat the pain itself. One of the principal benefits of pain treatment is reducing or eliminating the functional deficits caused by pain. It is these deficits that determine the medical necessity of pain treatment as balanced against the deficits induced by the pain treatment itself.

Medical science struggles to explain why chronic pain exists. What is its purpose? How has it survived the evolutionary process? How does it promote survival? It is common in professional pain literature to see a contrast between "good" acute pain that protects and promotes lives and "bad" chronic pain that protects nothing and promotes nothing. Acute pain protects us until healing is complete, but chronic pain persists indefinitely. Acute pain makes sense and chronic pain does not. Chronic pain is pain that persists beyond healing time. Perhaps chronic joint pain protects joints from further degeneration, but what is chronic back pain protecting us from, or chronic headaches? Diabetic neuropathic pain can be explained as a side effect of metabolic damage to our peripheral nerves, but what about fibromyalgia?

We can only escape from this paradox if we stop thinking of pain as a damage detection system and start thinking of it as a danger detection system. It takes a predictable amount of time to heal a broken femur, but an unpredictable amount of time to heal a broken heart. It may take a long time to heal a fractured pelvis, but not as long as it takes to heal from incest. For humans, the physical pain and social pain systems are built on top of each other. Evolution has expanded the simple physical pain modulation system of non-mammals into the complex physical and social pain modulation system of mammals, including rodents, primates, and humans.[7] The human system senses and modulates a broader sense of danger and creates a more complex and varied pain experience. This includes chronic pain conditions whose protective functions can be obscure. Pelvic pain may protect against further sexual activity in incest survivors, but the protective effects of back pain in survivors of physical abuse are not as clear.

Redefine the necessity to provide opioids for pain

Only through clear criteria for the medical necessity of pain treatment can we find a way to reconcile the simultaneous claims of opioid over-prescribing and under-prescribing found in the professional and popular literature.[8-10] With 5% of the world's population, the United States prescribes 80% of the opioids.[11] What is the proper amount of opioid prescribing? Opioid prescribing in the United States is down since 2012, but still remains at least double that in 1999. The Centers for Disease Control and Prevention has summarized recent prescribing data. In 2017, more than 17% of Americans had at least one opioid prescription filled, and the average was 3.4 prescriptions dispensed per patient. The average daily dose of opioids was over 45 mg of morphine or equivalent. The duration per prescription is still increasing, to an average of 18 days in 2017.[12] Counties vary widely in opioid prescribing, with higher-prescribing counties characterized by social features such as smaller cities or larger towns, a higher percentage of White residents, lower household income, and more people who are uninsured or unemployed. They are also characterized by these medical features: more dentists and primary care physicians per capita and more residents who have diabetes, arthritis, or a disability.[13] Opioid prescribing is driven by an array of medical and non-medical features of a patient's environment. Rates of manual labor, unemployment, and high school graduation have all shown associations with opioid prescribing.[14] Prescribing rates vary considerably among different physicians in the same emergency room.[15]

Determining the proper level of opioid prescribing is complex for many reasons. Among patients prescribed opioids for low back pain without significant evidence of opioid misuse in the past year, daily opioid use was prompted as strongly by negative emotions as by pain and provided relief of both negative emotions and pain. Among participants at high risk for opioid misuse, pain, but not negative emotions, was associated with higher opioid doses.[16] This defies our standard understanding of prescription opioid use for physical pain as proper use and prescription opioid use for negative emotions as improper abuse. However, this pattern of opioid use for both physical and social pain is to be expected if our account of pain, anxiety, and depression as homeostatic emotions presented in the previous chapter is accurate. Distressed patients feel both negative emotions and localized pain. They use and abuse opioids for both afflictions.

Pharmaceutical marketing and professional treatment guidelines have all urged opioid prescribers to focus on the treatment of physical pain rather than the treatment of those with emotional pain, as manifested in mental health and substance use disorders. These admonitions have failed completely. Patients with mental health and substance use disorders are more likely to be prescribed opioids, at higher doses, for longer periods of time.[17] *Given the evolutionary history and complex purposes of the human pain system, it is simply not possible to aim prescription opioids at physical pain only and not at the whole of human suffering, nor to distinguish exactly which of these is being treated.*

Our understanding of opioid abuse and addiction changes if we use the homeostatic emotions concept along with the salience network and danger detection ideas developed in the previous chapter. The homeostatic emotion idea sees pain as reflecting threats to homeostasis, including threats to bodily integrity or personal integrity. Classically, opioid addicts are said to start use of opioids to "get high" while legitimate patients use opioids for physical pain relief. But euphoria is a transient, nonuniversal, and imprecise understanding of the effect of opioids in addicts. More compelling are descriptions of a feeling of complete and profound safety after using heroin. Amanda Ryan-Carr, when she was quoted in the *New York Times*, explained about heroin: "It's like being hugged by Jesus."[18] For believers, only God can create this feeling of absolute safety. Given the high rates of neglect and trauma among heroin users that produce a chronic sense of danger, it is easy to understand how a feeling of total safety, once experienced, could be irresistible. In the same *New York Times* article about our opioid epidemic, Matt Statman from Michigan stated, "I remember feeling like I was exhaling from holding my breath for my whole life. Just intense relief from suffering."[18] As heroin takes effect, an unrelenting sense of danger disappears completely. Even as actual life falls apart, heroin's hug from God tells us we are absolutely safe. As described by Brandon from Pennsylvania, "It was like the high put on blinders to everything and made me not care about anything in the world, other than the heroin."[18] If pain perception is guided by the salience network, feelings of safety are an essential modifier of that perception. Opioids have long been reported to reduce pain affect more than pain intensity. Feelings of safety may thus be an important motivation for opioid use, misuse, and abuse.

One of the most perplexing and difficult aspects of determining the need for opioid pain treatment is that the use of opioid treatment for any significant length of time creates the need for more opioid treatment through opioid tolerance. Bioethicist Travis Rieder has described his experience with opioids following a motorcycle accident that crushed his foot and ankle.[19] After taking daily high-dose opioids for months exactly as prescribed by his doctors, he found himself unable to discontinue these opioids. When he tried to gradually reduce his dose, not only did he have the classic restlessness, insomnia, irritability, and flu-like symptoms of opioid withdrawal, but he also had more pain. It was unclear if this was his original injury pain (his foot was healing) or opioid-induced hyperalgesia. More importantly, as he reduced his opioids, for the first time in his life he "felt suddenly and immediately overwhelmed" and he became "truly miserable—abjectly and utterly miserable":

> The crying now brought with it darkness, and I would feel whatever peace I had managed to scrape together on that day slip away from me as the sadness descended. It came from anywhere or nowhere, and when it did come there was no stopping it . . . When the darkness swirled in, my mind

went to scary places. I began to genuinely mourn what had happened to me, and also believe that it meant the end of the happy life I had known before. I became convinced that I would never recover—not from the accident, not from the withdrawal.[19(p94)]

His doctors suggested he either get addiction services or resume his opioids. But he had no signs of addiction, for he had never misused his medication or taken extra medication and sincerely wanted to discontinue opioids. No one knew how to deal with his opioid dependence.

Iatrogenically induced opioid dependence may be among the most difficult aspects of determining the need for long-term opioid therapy. This has become a significant public health problem as clinicians and health systems have been trying to taper patients treated with opioids for years off dangerous high-dose opioid therapy. These tapers are intended to reduce the ongoing risks of overdose and addiction in these patients. Most patients who undergo gradual and supervised opioid tapers do well, without significant increase in pain.[20] But other patients, who have abrupt or unsupervised tapers, or who simply have been on continuous high-dose opioids for years, may have severe difficulties with opioid taper. Contrary to conventional understanding, these withdrawal symptoms may not be simply "physical" or temporary as is thought to be typical of opioid withdrawal when physically dependent. Pain may return at the original injury site.[21] Despair, hopelessness, and suicidal ideation may appear and persist for long periods. Some of these patients may never be able to discontinue opioids. This may be due to the development of complex persistent opioid dependence, a condition that we have described in the scientific literature.[22] Luckily, buprenorphine appears to help many of these patients.[23]

Unwinding mechanical clinical pain

Mental pain is less dramatic than physical pain, but it is more common and also more hard to bear. The frequent attempt to conceal mental pain increases the burden: it is easier to say "My tooth is aching" than to say "My heart is broken."

C. S. Lewis

The moral necessity of medical pain treatment

One layer deeper than the *medical* necessity of opioid pain treatment is the *moral* necessity of opioid pain treatment. The clearest and most succinct statement of this comes from Sidney Wanzer in the *New England Journal of Medicine* in 1989: "The proper dose of pain medication is the dose that is sufficient to relieve pain and suffering ... To allow a patient to experience unbearable pain or suffering is unethical medical practice."[24(p845)] Wanzer made this argument in the context of palliative care, but it is the same argument that has been made in chronic pain care.[25,26] We have argued in the last chapter that this argument for opioid relief is based on the idea that chronic pain is a form of *innocent suffering*. By innocent suffering we mean suffering imposed upon the person, suffering that they did not deserve, could not prevent, and are powerless to escape. And we have argued that this moral status of chronic pain is based on a *mechanical model* of chronic pain causation. In its classical formulation, the patient as person is not included in this model. In its expanded biopsychosocial model, psychological and social modifiers of the biologically caused pain are included in the model. When these modifiers are addressed through cognitive–behavioral therapy, the aim is generally to reduce the suffering and disability associated with chronic pain, rather than reducing or eliminating the pain itself. Pain psychology positions itself as a supplement to medical pain treatment, not as a replacement for it. This means that it has not directly challenged our culture's image of pain as innocent suffering.

Modern medicine sees pain, like disease, as arising within our body. This pain attacks us from its place *inside the body, but outside our mind, outside our self, outside our soul*. We call upon clinicians to relieve us of this pain, which we do not deserve. This pain produces suffering, but is not itself suffering. Pain is produced by mechanisms in the body that medical professionals can assess, understand, and treat. This is unlike suffering, which includes all the psychological, cultural, and religious complexity of human life. Within this modern medical perspective, it makes sense to separate localized, physical pain from the rest of human suffering because we can understand this pain and control it. We understand its mechanical causation and its surgical and pharmacological treatment. We construe this medicalized pain as inessential suffering that can be controlled by impersonal treatments that attack the pain and leave the person alone. This has helped us free pain of its deep historical roots in deserved punishment. We discourage patients from asking Job's question to the God of the Old Testament, "*Why* am I in pain?", because we would prefer to talk about *how* they are in pain. This is because we see this physical pain as inessential suffering that we can relieve with medical tools, not as essential suffering that must be understood and accepted as part of who we are as individuals and as humans.

Our modern efforts to control pain (like anesthesia for surgery) have thankfully shifted the boundary between pain that must be accepted and pain that can be relieved. This is surely an important part of human and medical progress. The reductions achieved in premature death and uncontrolled pain are among our society's proudest achievements. But we have learned in recent years that not all deaths are premature. Most now agree that it is ethical and humane to accept some deaths. Most agree that doing all we can to prevent all deaths can lead to great harm and little benefit. In this book, we have made a parallel argument about pain. Seeking to eliminate all chronic pain by medical means (generally opioids) has brought great harm and little benefit. Some acceptance of pain into the flow of human life is necessary and prudent. Not all pain can be isolated from the rest of human suffering and conquered with medical tools.

Reuniting pain and suffering, mechanism and meaning

Your patient, Daniel Perkins, has challenged you: "Don't you believe I am in pain? Don't you believe I deserve relief?" What if instead he had asked: "Do you not believe I am suffering? Do you not believe that I deserve relief?" By speaking of suffering rather than pain, Daniel has shifted his question and the kind of request he is making of you. This request is less medical, more personal and individualized. In using the term "suffering," he portrays his condition as less passive, less mechanical, and perhaps less innocent, for modern patients see suffering as more within their control than pain. If Daniel's suffering arose from grief, or loneliness, or poverty, or depression, we would expect him to play a role in overcoming it. Calling Daniel's plight "suffering" rather than "pain" calls less for medication and more for his personal engagement. Pain is medical but suffering is not, at least not completely.

Palliative care has succeeded in bringing the assessment and treatment of suffering back into the modern hospital after its long banishment. In his famous 1982 article "The Nature of Suffering and the Goals of Medicine," internist Eric Cassell argues that:

> The question of suffering and its relation to organic illness has rarely been addressed in the medical literature.... A distinction based on clinical observations is made between suffering and physical distress. *Suffering is experienced by persons, not merely by bodies*, and has its source in challenges that threaten the intactness of the person as a complex social and psychological entity. Suffering can include physical pain but is by no means limited to it.[27(p642)] (emphasis added)

Cassell argues that suffering happens to persons. We are arguing that pain also happens to persons, not just their bodies. Cassell further argues that the relief of suffering must be considered equal to the cure of disease as a core obligation of "a medical profession that is truly dedicated to the care of the sick."[27(p642)] Our "failure to understand the nature of suffering can result in medical intervention that ... not only fails to relieve suffering but becomes a source of suffering itself."[27(p642)] But as pain relief became a higher priority for medicine throughout the 1980s and 1990s, somehow its separation from suffering became more marked. *We depersonalized pain to destigmatize it.* In so doing we unleashed opioid treatment, with all its promise and peril.

We privilege pain as a form of physical suffering. Like acute pain and disease, we consider this chronic pain to be innocent suffering caused by objective damage: "You did nothing to bring this on yourself." Parallel and corollary to this passive and innocent suffering is a form of pain-specific relief, opioid painkillers. We prescribe opioids to "kill" the pain and leave the person alone. As our patients say to us, "Don't give me any of your mind-altering (e.g., antidepressant) drugs; just take away my pain!" These patients do not want to see their pain and suffering as wrapped up with their personhood. Their pain is something produced by their body, and it is medicine's business to make it go away. This is a serious misunderstanding of pain and of opioids that has helped lead us into our opioid epidemic.

Pain and suffering are not as distinct as our patients believe, nor as distinct as the mechanical model of nociception and pain perception would have clinicians believe. It is not true that the aversive sensation of pain arrives in the brain where it is perceived and produces emotional suffering. Pain clinicians (both physicians and psychologists) often try to destigmatize discussion of emotions and suffering for patients with chronic pain by portraying them as "reasonable reactions" to the aversive experience of pain. It is certainly true that pain is usually a distressing experience. But to separate suffering from pain as an emotional reaction impoverishes our understanding of pain and its role in human life. Human pain is as complex as human suffering. Our interpersonal environment shapes not only our emotional reaction to pain, but also its very intensity, extent, and duration.

Pain and suffering actually have a bidirectional relationship. Pain causes suffering, but suffering also causes pain. Psychological trauma, posttraumatic stress disorder, depression, and anxiety are all more common in patients with chronic pain. Prospective studies show that these forms of suffering often *precede* the development of chronic pain.[28-30] Abnormalities of our endogenous opioid system are seen in chronic pain and in major depression.[31,32] This bidirectional relationship is consistent with our understanding of pain, anxiety, and depression as protective homeostatic emotions. But it is not consistent with our traditional understanding of suffering as an emotional reaction to pain. You cannot simply tell Daniel that his pain "is all in his head." His pain is not imaginary; he cannot simply wish it away.

On the other hand, suffering in patients who experience chronic pain, anxiety, or depression is not entirely innocent, because there is always something they can do to improve the course of their condition. Patients must participate in treatment. Passive submission to treatment is not adequate, just as it is not adequate for other forms of suffering like grief, depression, or loneliness. Passive submission to treatment is also not adequate for chronic diseases like diabetes. While patients are not responsible for having chronic pain (backward-looking responsibility), they are responsible for participating in recovery (forward-looking responsibility). Reducing all forms of suffering is relevant to recovery from chronic pain. It is not true that pain must be reduced first, before recovery is possible. Patients' habits, beliefs, behaviors, and social relationships are all relevant to recovery, but not under direct control of a treating healthcare professional. The recovery and exercise of agency by patients is crucial to their recovery from chronic pain. Social reactivation and physical reactivation are among the most reliable treatments for both chronic pain and depression.[33,34]

It is not true that the sensory aspects of pain invariably precede and determine the motor aspects of pain. There is no simple linear path from pain experience to pain behavior, especially in chronic pain. Patient action is both a means and an end for chronic pain care.[35] Patient activation is an important strategy in chronic pain rehabilitation. This rehabilitation need not focus on decreasing pain, because pain reduction is not a prerequisite for successful rehabilitation.[36] Multiple converging lines of research suggest that expanding opportunities for and confidence in purposive action by patients with chronic pain may be a potent means for reducing pain salience and thereby reducing pain intensity.[37] Part of this effort is convincing patients that it is safe to move, safe to take initiative, safe to connect with other people.

Patient action does not simply occur in the face of pain of specific intensity; rather, this action may itself reduce pain salience and the pain-related disruption of the patient's life. By making the patient's investment in life stronger, by helping them rediscover the passions and the values that make each a unique person, and by directing our treatment efforts toward the facilitation of this rediscovery, we can lessen the disruptive effect of pain. When patient action is the central goal of treatment, clinical interactions and interventions are directed at restoring patients' capacity to define and achieve life goals through action. In chronic illness, the patient must act as the agent through which healthcare is delivered and by which health is achieved.[38] Pain clinicians need to elicit and promote patients' life goals, as they provide the energy for patient action and are the proper focus for treatment. Penney Cowan and the American Chronic Pain Association identify one of the crucial challenges in chronic pain management as "making the journey from patient to person." Restoring the capacity for meaningful action is what transforms someone with chronic pain from a patient into a person.

Redefine the moral necessity of pain treatment

This goal of personhood redefines the moral necessity of pain treatment. Consider an account of our current understanding of the moral necessity of opioid pain treatment in a 2019 report by Human Rights Watch on the U.S. opioid situation entitled *Not Allowed to Be Compassionate* (Figure 9.3).[39] Their report begins with the case of Maria Higginbotham, a 43-year-old regional bank manager. Her diagnosis is listed as "an aggressive form of

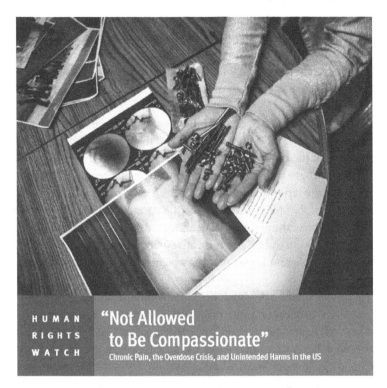

Figure 9.3. Cover of the Human Rights Watch report *Not Allowed to Be Compassionate*

degenerative disc disorder" for which she has had multiple back surgeries with instrumentation that has left her with "adhesive arachnoiditis." She has tried and failed many treatments, but now uses oral opioid medication, an intrathecal opioid pump, and opioid patches, which allow her to do household chores and care for her grandchildren. Then, in response to the Centers for Disease Control opioid guidelines that specify when opioid doses become unsafe, her pain doctor announces that he will reduce her opioids by 75%. He states that he fears legal liability if he does not taper her opioids. As her opioids are tapered by a third, her pain escalates and she loses 70 pounds and becomes bedridden.

The Human Rights Watch report, based on interviews with 86 patients, providers, and officials in Tennessee and Washington, argues that:

[U]nder international human rights standards, actions taken to combat the overdose epidemic should take the needs of chronic pain patients into account. The government should seek to avoid harming chronic pain patients: some patients still have a *legitimate need* for these medications.[39(p2)] (emphasis added)

These patients are contrasted with patients where opioids "may not be benefitting them [who] should be weaned off them safely."[39(p15,21,23)] We are cautioned that these patients should not be "characterized as 'drug seekers,' rather than people with serious health problems that require treatment."[39] Throughout the report there is a focus on "chronic pain patients who have a *medical need* for opioid analgesics."[39] The report concludes by calling for implementation of the multimodal treatment advocated in the National Pain Strategy and also an end to "administrative practices that arbitrarily interfere with the ability of chronic pain patients who need opioid analgesics to access them."[39]

We do not doubt Ms. Higginbotham's pain and suffering. She has received many surgical and pharmacological treatments for her back pain that have not helped her and likely have harmed her. She has been on high-dose opioid therapy for many years and now is undergoing an involuntary and rapid opioid taper. The medical profession is responsible for selling her these treatments and now for withdrawing them. It may be necessary to continue her opioid treatment for the rest of her life. But her need for continued opioids is not simply due to her original back pain problem; it is also due to the surgical and especially pharmacological treatments she has received. Here, medical mistakes lead to iatrogenic harm that then lead to the demand for more medical treatments. As we have seen in the case of Travis Rieder above, opioid treatment creates the need for more opioid treatment through opioid tolerance and opioid dependence. This dependence may be a "legitimate need" for opioid treatment at this point in her back pain care, even though it is hard to see Ms. Higginbotham's surgical and medication treatment as successful.

Due to her history of failed back pain treatments, Ms. Higginbotham is currently not a good case in which to examine the general right to pain relief or moral necessity of pain care. Our current duties are tied to her failed treatments. The moral necessity of surgical or opioid treatment for her degenerative disc disorder is doubtful. Neither of these treatments has documented efficacy for this condition, which is present in many older adults with no back pain. We are not given details of the early stages of her back pain condition or treatment, so it is difficult to know what were the viable treatment alternatives.

We do know that there is a natural antagonism between professional treatments for chronic pain and patients' chronic pain self-management efforts. One naturally substitutes for the other, though it is possible to pursue both. As Ivan Illich argued in his famous "Killing Pain" chapter of *Medical Nemesis*, once a professional medical treatment for pain is available (e.g., epidural infusion for labor pain), self-managing and tolerating pain ceases to be noble and becomes just stupid.[40] Why endure labor pain when there is a safe and effective treatment for it? The answer, as any home birth advocate might tell you, is that there is more to the birth experience than pain, and epidurals affect more aspects of that experience than just pain.[41]

The right to pain relief, and the moral assessment of pain as innocent suffering it is based on, as well as the mechanical model of pain that underlies all of these, needs to be dismantled if we are to avoid placing more patients into the sorry situation of Ms. Higginbotham. Chronic illness is more complex, both causally and morally, than acute illness. There is no clear separation between the person and the chronic illness, as is characteristic of acute illness. When pneumonia resolves, one goes back to being the same person as before the pneumonia. This is not true for diabetes or for chronic pain. It is not possible to have good care for one's diabetes without changing one's beliefs, behaviors, and habits. The same is true for chronic pain.

In 1996, the American Pain Society and the American Academy of Pain Medicine jointly adopted a consensus statement "On the Use of Opioids in the Treatment of Chronic Pain." This statement was published in 1997 and adopted by the Federation of State Medical Boards as Model Guidelines for the Use of Controlled Substances for the Treatment of Pain in 1998.[42] As David Haddox pointed out in his 1998 American Academy of Pain Medicine presidential address, the most important part of these guidelines is the first sentence of the preamble, which states: "The (name of state Board) recognizes that principles of quality medical practice dictate that the people of the State of (name of state) *have access to appropriate and effective pain relief.*"[43] Haddox makes the argument that these guidelines are not only about opioids, or about controlled substances generally, but about the right of pain relief in medical practice. We agree that this right to pain relief goes deeper than opioid prescribing. But it provides the fertile ground within which the opioid epidemic grew.

America has the worst opioid epidemic in the world, at least in part because it has one of the weakest and most medicalized social safety nets of all advanced economies. We don't provide Americans much protection against suffering unless it is deemed medical. That is because we give moral priority to medical suffering. This moral priority is stronger in America than in other countries. This is one reason why our opioid epidemic is worse than that in other countries. Our medical safety net is also famously incomplete, but still offers more support for medical conditions than for employment, housing, education, and childcare. This medical safety net requires that suffering be associated with a medical diagnosis to be eligible for services.[44] This has helped separate pain from suffering. This is another deep root of our opioid epidemic.

Recently, Donald Berwick, MD, former administrator for the Center for Medicare and Medicaid Services and former president of the Institute for Healthcare Improvement, has called for greater attention to the "moral determinants of health."[45(p226)] This means not just identifying the social determinants of health but also developing programs, and especially health services, to address them. He quotes Sir Michael Marmot, a pioneer in research into the social determinants of health, in noting that "fairness" and "social solidarity" are the most important health determinants to address.[45] In fact, economists Case and Deaton point to deficits in fairness and social solidarity as the primary causes of the opioid-related "deaths of despair" that they discovered and described. We are, therefore, supportive of efforts to improve fairness and solidarity as ways to reduce both chronic pain and the opioid epidemic. But among "the first-order elements of a morally guided campaign for better health" that Berwick lists is the "realization in statute of health care as a human right in the US."[45] "This agenda includes, but is by no means restricted to, ensuring care for patients with illness and disease, no matter how they acquired their conditions."[45] Here we must differ: The United States must care for its *citizens*, not just for its patients with illness and disease. It should not be necessary to be diagnosed with an illness or disease to qualify for support or mercy in times of need. We select illness and disease as blameless afflictions that deserve our care. But it is not necessary to medicalize pain and suffering to address their roots in lack of fairness and solidarity. Berwick himself acknowledges that healthcare is not the most important determinant of health in a society. Mending "the fabric of communities upon which health depends," as he puts it, will require other means than medical techniques or medical practitioners.

Based on his horrific experience with opioids, Travis Rieder concludes: "We all need to foster a different relationship with pain and develop a different understanding of medicine—what it does and doesn't owe us, and what we should expect from our doctors."[19(p257)] We have progressively medicalized our social safety net and required medical certification of inability to work. Pain is at the center of the medicalization of unemployment as disability.[46] Yet, for patients with pain, the distinction between "can't work" and "won't work" is *not* a scientific distinction.[47,48] Even if we were able to verify and quantify the amount of pain experienced by a patient, we would not be able to determine if this made it impossible, or difficult, or just undesirable to work. Pain's effect on the ability to work can only be understood in the context of a complex and varied set of personal incentives. The issue is not whether this pain is "real" (associated with identifiable medical cause). Pain has unmatched moral authority in our culture to justify disability and to warrant opioid treatment. We will not be able to address the opioid crisis until we begin to question this unique status of pain as passive and innocent suffering that warrants a medical response.

Unwinding the social war on pain: minimizing pain and suffering

Pain makes me grow. Growing is what I want. Therefore, for me pain is pleasure.

Arnold Schwarzenegger

Daniel Perkins, part 2

You agree to prescribe Daniel a slowly decreasing dose of oxycodone over a series of weekly clinic visits. Over the past month's visits, you have gotten the chance to talk to Daniel about more than pills and pain levels. He told you about the time he was suicidal and almost killed himself by throwing himself off a bridge. You ask if his pain was at its worst at that time. He says, "Yes, it was." Then he goes on to say that this was right after his estranged daughter confronted him about his years of heavy drinking when she was young and he couldn't be bothered with making her food or taking her to school. She told him that she did not want to see him ever again. That was the most intense pain he had ever felt. It was more than he could stand, and so he walked toward the tall bridge over the freeway to throw himself off. But before he got to the bridge, he passed a young woman walking her dog and sobbing. He tried to reach out to her, but she stepped away. At that moment, he realized that his daughter needed him alive, even if she did not realize it. Now she seemed more important than his pain.

As we discussed in Chapter 1, our modern medical effort to eliminate pain takes place within the general social effort to reduce pain and suffering to a minimum. This is the task that the French *philosophes* of the 18th-century Enlightenment, and the English utilitarians who followed them in the 19th century, set for the secular society that they had wrested out of the hands of the Catholic Church. While the Church justified pain as promoting eternal salvation, the utilitarians focused on reducing pain to promote human flourishing during this lifetime. In our secular age, we are no longer focused on a life beyond this one. Modern secularism focuses on our current life as the only possible source of meaning and satisfaction. Is this general social goal to reduce pain and suffering relevant to the opioid epidemic? It is not nearly as directly relevant as medical pain measures and pain therapies, but our utilitarian focus on minimizing suffering provides the social context out of which medical and public health policies grow.

Secularism no longer looks to God and the Church to tell us what is true and how to have a happy life. As a largely secularized culture, we look to science for ways to maximize our happiness. This is how we determine the best way to maximize fame and fortune. Modern science is based on the authority of the objective point of view. This "view from nowhere" (to use Thomas Nagel's phrase[49]) is authoritative because it is unbiased, not limited to a particular point of view, and can therefore claim to generate universal truths. In our modern perspective, a priority is given to "the neutral grasp of things" for both facts and values. For utilitarians, the right action is the one that will produce the most pleasure and the least pain for everyone. Science can tell us which action this is. Not only scientific facts about how to make something happen, but also facts about the utility or happiness produced by an action, are best apprehended from a neutral point of view. We have secularized this neutral point of view from which the truth about the balance of pain and pleasure is apprehended. It is now objectivity rather than God that ensures this view is true. We have thus removed God from our notion of society, but not the impartial God-like view of the world.

Utilitarianism takes a detached view of maximizing pleasure and minimizing pain, concerned more with the final balance of pleasure and pain than the path we used to get there. This makes it a powerfully simple perspective on policy, but a dangerously truncated view of human life and personal aspiration. Some experts have denied that the most pleasurable and least painful human life is the best human life. To make this point, philosopher Robert Nozick proposed his famous thought experiment about the "experience machine."[50] Nozick asks us to imagine a machine that could give us whatever pleasurable experience we might want. When hooked up to this device, people believe they are loving, working, or eating and have the satisfaction associated with these activities, but they are actually doing none of them. Despite its efficiency in producing well-being, few would choose this experience machine over a life of choice and activity, even if these activities did not reliably produce well-being. This is because, Nozick argues, we want to actually do things, not just have the experience of doing them: "It is only because we first want to do the actions that we want the experiences of doing them."[50(p43)] Utilitarianism can seduce us with its passive ideal of maximized pleasure and minimized pain, but it is not an image of a satisfying, meaningful, or rewarding human life. As philosopher Martha Nussbaum comments: "In short, the utilitarian metric seems to care about people, but it doesn't care about them all that deeply, and its commitment to a single metric effaces a great deal about how people seek and find value in their lives."[51(p52–53)] Contrary to the utilitarian view, a pain-free life is not a good life.

Nozick's point is that humans don't just want the most pleasant life; we want to participate, to achieve, to overcome obstacles. For this reason, Arnold Schwarzenegger and Friedrich Nietzsche are willing to tolerate pain, even to invite it. "No pain" does not work as a goal for life. The goal of "no pain" says nothing about what you want to do and be with your life. A perspective on life that only tallies pleasure and pain, or more broadly happiness and suffering, omits the active aspect of life. It omits the fact that we are not only consumers in life but also agents.

Beyond pain reduction to capability promotion

The shortcomings of pain minimization for individual human lives can be seen when this metric is applied to societies. Development economist and Nobel laureate Amartya Sen has advocated moving away from the balance of happiness and suffering, otherwise known as "welfare," as the primary index of development for societies toward one based on capabilities. Sen developed the concept of capability in his famous Tanner Lectures, "Equality of What?", where he argued the most important equality for a just society is neither objective economic resources (e.g., gross domestic product) nor subjective well-being (e.g., welfare or more pleasure than pain), but the concrete capabilities and functionings of its citizens.[52] Functionings are the means by which it is possible "to do and to be" what one wishes. Even more basic than functionings are capabilities, which concern the person's ability to function. One example of an important functioning is voting. The capability of literacy provides the ability to vote in a meaningful and effective way.

One important capability is to pursue and promote one's own health. In the case of pain management, this capability includes the ability to self-manage one's pain. Jennifer Ruger argues that health policy and bioethics often neglect this "health capability" by thinking that health is only provided through professional healthcare.[53] She argues that both health consequences (e.g., pain levels) and health agency (e.g., capacity to manage pain) are important goals for health policy. The populace should be provided not only with health, but also the means to address and improve its health. *Where health comes from is important.* In other words, the means by which health goals, such as improved functioning, are achieved is as important as the achievement itself: "Health capability integrates health outcomes and health agency."[(p45)] It concerns both the "what" and the "how" of health. In the case of pain, it concerns both whether pain relief is achieved and how it is achieved. It concerns whether it is the patient or the professional who is providing pain relief.

Rewinding pain back into our vision of a complete human life

The cure for pain is in the pain.

Rumi

The utilitarians' arguments in favor of minimizing pain and suffering can be very persuasive in their appeal to modern common sense: Who wants more suffering? But then we must consider Charles Taylor's question, "Is that all there is? There seems to be no room for generous action, heroism, the warrior virtues, a higher sensibility; or else for a real dedication to humanity, a more demanding ethic of sacrifice."[54(p545)] There are traces of interest in some good beyond human flourishing in concerns about global warming and mass extinctions. But these still lie at the margins of our culture, which is mainly focused on human survival and comfort.

Modern medicine is one of the finest fruits of the Enlightenment, helping us reduce premature death and acute illness and cast off the fatalism of the medieval period. As historian Peter Gay summarizes, "Medicine was the most highly visible and the most heartening index of general improvement: nothing was after all better calculated to buoy up men's feeling about life than growing hope for life itself."[55(p145)] In addition to reducing premature mortality, modern medicine has helped move the boundary between essential (or inescapable) pain and inessential (or treatable) pain. We are still afraid of dying from painful cancer, but not as fearful and powerless as we once were. We have anesthesia for surgery and triptans for migraine headaches.

Opioids are part of the medical armaments that have shifted the boundary between pain that can be controlled and pain that must be accepted. During the most messianic early days of opioid liberalization, we heard claims that wider prescribing of opioids would lower the total suffering of society. This has not happened. Considering opioid overdose deaths, addiction, and all the related social chaos, we believe that opioid liberalization has increased the total suffering, at least of Americans.

So what is the right balance? How much pain control is too much pain control? Pain and suffering are inescapable, even valuable, aspects of human life. Any quest for their elimination will distort life. The goal of a "pain-free life" is not a good one. The utilitarians were mistaken about this. This is because pain and pleasure are not opposites and do not exclude each other; they can increase or decrease together. Friedrich Nietzsche asks us: "Did you ever say yes to all pleasure? Oh my friends, then you also said yes to all pain. All things are linked, entwined, in love with one another."(*The Gay Science,* p84) When we shut down the capacity for pain, we shut down the capacity for pleasure. This is consistent with what we know about how opioids influence our brain's reward system. It is also consistent with the best advice of saints and scholars. As Franz Kafka (Figure 9.4) cautions us, "You can hold yourself back from the sufferings of the world, that is something you are free to do and it accords with your nature, but perhaps this very holding back is the one suffering you could avoid."

In our modern era, we are haunted not by evil demons, but by meaninglessness. We are less afraid of being punished than of being set adrift without a moral compass. We have gotten quite good at answering the question concerning *how* pain is caused and treated, but we have gotten quite bad

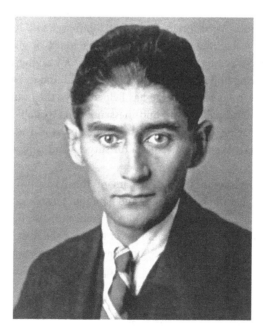

Figure 9.4. Franz Kafka
https://commons.wikimedia.org/wiki/File:Kafka.jpg. (Wikipedia public domain)

at answering the question about *why* we should suffer pain. We struggle to come up with a good reason for suffering. As Japanese author Yukio Mishima said, "We live in an age in which there is no heroic death." With no reason to die, we may also have no reason to live. What is worth dying for? What is worth living for? What is worth suffering for? Human meaning is born in the answers to these questions.

References

1. Price R. *A Whole New Life: An Illness and a Healing.* Scribner; 1995.
2. Ballantyne JC, Sullivan MD. Intensity of chronic pain—the wrong metric? *N Engl J Med.* 2015;373:2098–2099.
3. Krebs EE, Lorenz KA, Bair MJ, et al. Development and initial validation of the PEG, a three-item scale assessing pain intensity and interference. *J Gen Intern Med.* 2009;24:733–738.
4. Joint Commission on Accreditation of Healthcare Organizations; National Pharmaceutical Council. *Pain: Current Understanding of Assessment, Management and Treatments.* National Pharmaceutical Council; 2001.
5. R3 Report Issue 11: Pain Assessment and Management Standards for Hospitals, The Joint Commission. 2018. https://www.jointcommission.org/standards/r3-report/r3-report-issue-11-pain-assessment-and-management-standards-for-hospitals/#.Y08PGHbMKUk. Accessed 10-18-22.
6. Dahlhamer J, Lucas J, Zelaya C, et al. Prevalence of chronic pain and high-impact chronic pain among adults—United States, 2016. *MMWR Morb Mortal Wkly Rep.* 2018;67:1001–1006.
7. Eisenberger NI. Social pain and the brain: controversies, questions, and where to go from here. *Annu Rev Psychol.* 2015;66:601–629.
8. Volkow ND, Jones EB, Einstein EB, Wargo EM. Prevention and treatment of opioid misuse and addiction: a review. *JAMA Psychiatry.* 2019;76:208–216.
9. Ballantyne JC. Opioids for the treatment of chronic pain: mistakes made, lessons learned, and future directions. *Anesth Analg.* 2017;125:1769–1778.
10. Compton WM, Boyle M, Wargo E. Prescription opioid abuse: problems and responses. *Prev Med.* 2015;80:5–9.
11. Degenhardt L, Grebeley J, Stone J, et al. Global patterns of opioid use and dependence: harms to populations, interventions, and future action. *Lancet.* 2019;394:1560–1579.

12. Centers for Disease Control and Prevention. Vital Signs: Opioid Painkiller Prescribing. July 2014. https://www.cdc.gov/vitalsigns/opioid-prescribing/index.html

13. Guy GP, Jr., Zhang K, Schieber LZ, et al. County-level opioid prescribing in the United States, 2015 and 2017. *JAMA Intern Med.* 2019;179(4):574–576.

14. Paulozzi LJ, Strickler GK, Kreiner PW, Koris CM. Controlled substance prescribing patterns—Prescription Behavior Surveillance System, eight states, 2013. *MMWR Surveill Summ.* 2015;64:1–14.

15. Barnett ML, Olenski AR, Jena AB. Opioid-prescribing patterns of emergency physicians and risk of long-term use. *N Engl J Med.* 2017;376:663–673.

16. Carpenter RW, Lane SP, Bruehl S, Trull TJ. Concurrent and lagged associations of prescription opioid use with pain and negative affect in the daily lives of chronic pain patients. *J Consult Clin Psychol.* 2019;87:872–886.

17. Sullivan MD. Depression effects on long-term prescription opioid use, abuse, and addiction. *Clin J Pain.* 2018;34:878–884.

18. Sinha S. A visual journey through addiction. *New York Times*, December 18, 2018.

19. Rieder T. *In Pain.* Harper Collins; 2019.

20. Sullivan MD, Turner JA, DiLodovico C, et al. Prescription opioid taper support for outpatients with chronic pain: a randomized controlled trial. *J Pain.* 2017;18(3):308–318.

21. Rieb LM, DeBeck K, Hayashi K, et al. Withdrawal-associated injury site pain prevalence and correlates among opioid-using people who inject drugs in Vancouver, Canada. *Drug Alcohol Depend.* 2020;216:108242.

22. Ballantyne JC, Sullivan MD, Koob GF. Refractory dependence on opioid analgesics. *Pain.* 2019;160(12):2655–2660.

23. Manhapra A, Arias AJ, Ballantyne JC. The conundrum of opioid tapering in long-term opioid therapy for chronic pain: a commentary. *Subst Abus.* 2018;39:152–161.

24. Wanzer SH, Federman DD, Adelstein SJ, et al. The physician's responsibility toward hopelessly ill patients: a second look. *N Engl J Med.* 1989;320:844–849.

25. Portenoy RK. Appropriate use of opioids for persistent non-cancer pain. *Lancet.* 2004;364:739–740.

26. Passik SD, Weinreb HJ. Managing chronic nonmalignant pain: overcoming obstacles to the use of opioids. *Adv Ther.* 2000;17:70–83.

27. Cassell EJ. The nature of suffering and the goals of medicine. *N Engl J Med.* 1982;306:639–645.

28. Katon W, Egan K, Miller D. Chronic pain: lifetime psychiatric diagnoses and family history. *Am J Psychiatry*. 1985;142:1156–1160.

29. Anda RF, Felitti VJ, Bremner JD, et al. The enduring effects of abuse and related adverse experiences in childhood: a convergence of evidence from neurobiology and epidemiology. *Eur Arch Psychiatry Clin Neurosci*. 2006;256:174–186.

30. Anda R, Tietjen G, Schulman E, et al. Adverse childhood experiences and frequent headaches in adults. *Headache*. 2010;50:1473–1481.

31. Schrepf A, Harper DE, Harte SE, et al. Endogenous opioidergic dysregulation of pain in fibromyalgia: a PET and fMRI study. *Pain*. 2016;157:2217–2225.

32. Light SN, Bieliauskas LA, Zubieta JK. "Top-down" mu-opioid system function in humans: mu-opioid receptors in ventrolateral prefrontal cortex mediate the relationship between hedonic tone and executive function in major depressive disorder. *J Neuropsychiatry Clin Neurosci*. 2017;29(4):357–364.

33. Geneen LJ, Moore RA, Clarke C, et al. Physical activity and exercise for chronic pain in adults: an overview of Cochrane Reviews. *Cochrane Database Syst Rev*. 2017;4:CD011279.

34. Kvam S, Kleppe CL, Nordhus IH, Hovland A. Exercise as a treatment for depression: a meta-analysis. *J Affect Disord*. 2016;202:67–86.

35. Sullivan MD, Vowles KE. Patient action: as means and end for chronic pain care. *Pain*. 2017;158:1405–1407.

36. Vowles KE, Witkiewitz K, Levell J, et al. Are reductions in pain intensity and pain-related distress necessary? An analysis of within-treatment change trajectories in relation to improved functioning following interdisciplinary acceptance and commitment therapy for adults with chronic pain. *J Consult Clin Psychol*. 2017;85:87–98.

37. Kucyi A, Davis KD. The neural code for pain: from single-cell electrophysiology to the dynamic pain connectome. *Neuroscientist*. 2017;23(4):397–414.

38. Sullivan MD. *Patient as Agent of Health and Health Care*. Oxford University Press; 2017.

39. Human Rights Watch. *Not Allowed to Be Compassionate: Chronic Pain, Overdose Crisis, and Unintended Harms in the US*. Human Rights Watch; 2019.

40. Illich I. *Medical Nemesis: The Expropriation of Health*. Pantheon Books; 1976.

41. Wax JR, Lucas FL, Lamont M, et al. Maternal and newborn outcomes in planned home birth vs planned hospital births: a metaanalysis. *Am J Obstet Gynecol*. 2010;203:243.

42. American Academy of Pain Medicine and the American Pain Society. The use of opioids for the treatment of chronic pain. Clin J Pain. 1997;13:6–8.

43. Haddox JD. American Academy of Pain Medicine president's message: total pain care—new concept? Clin J Pain. 1998;14:280–281.

44. Bradley EH, Taylor LA. *The American Health Care Paradox: Why Spending More Is Getting Us Less*. Public Affairs Press; 2013.

45. Berwick DM. Moral determinants of health. *JAMA*. 2020;324:225–226.

46. Teasell RW, Bombardier C. Employment-related factors in chronic pain and chronic pain disability. *Clin J Pain*. 2001;17:S39–S45.

47. Mather L, Kärkkäinen S, Narusyte J, et al. Sick leave due to back pain, common mental disorders and disability pension: common genetic liability. *Eur J Pain*. 2020;24(10):1892–1901.

48. Mather L, Ropponen A, Mittendorfer-Rutz E, et al. Health, work and demographic factors associated with a lower risk of work disability and unemployment in employees with lower back, neck and shoulder pain. *BMC Musculoskelet Disord*. 2019;20:622.

49. Nagel T. *The View from Nowhere*. Oxford University Press; 1986.

50. Nozick R. *Anarchy, State, and Utopia*. Basic Books; 1974: p. 43.

51. Nussbaum, Martha. *Creating capabilities: the human development approach*. Cambridge, Massachusetts: The Belknap Press of Harvard University Press; 2011. ISBN 9780674050549.

52. Sen A. Equality of what? In: McMurrin SM, ed. *The Tanner Lectures on Human Values* (Volume 4). 2nd ed. Cambridge University Press; 2010:195–220.

53. Ruger JP. Health capability: conceptualization and operationalization. *Am J Public Health*. 2010;100:41–49.

54. Taylor C. *A Secular Age*. Harvard University Press; 2007.

55. Gay P. *The Enlightenment: An Interpretation*. Knopf; 1969.

10
Epilogue: Clinician's perspective
Dr. Clark's tale

It is an ordinary day. I arrive in the office at 7 a.m. and look through my patient list. I have 3 new patients and 12 follow-ups. I look at the names of the follow-up patients and realize that 3 of them are patients with chronic pain that I always dread seeing. I dread seeing them because they are in so much distress, yet nothing I have done seems to help them. They are angry and not satisfied with the care I provide. When they leave my office, I feel both irritable and worn out. I went into medicine to help people. Medical school taught me to problem solve, to arrive at a diagnosis, and to offer treatment. It means a lot to me when my patients get better and are grateful to me for helping them. But I know that these 3 patients will leave my office in as much distress as when they arrived—maybe even more. This upsets me and makes me wonder if I have the right skills to be a primary care doctor.

There's Annie Smith. She has been my patient for 9 years, since she moved to town. She is 44 and has fibromyalgia and diabetes. She hasn't worked since she was 30, and pain is her reason for not working. She lives alone and has 3 adult children whom she raised as a single mother. She was already on opioids when I took over her care. Over the past 9 years, her pain and distress have increased, despite my increasing her opioid dose, trying all the non-opioid medications I know, and encouraging her to exercise and to find something meaningful to do with her life. Every time I see her, she wants a higher opioid dose. That's the reason she comes in. She tells me that she was doing really well on the last dose, but now it doesn't seem to work as well, so she needs more. Sometimes we have a battle and she leaves without a sanctioned dose increase, very unhappy with me. Sometimes I give in and increase her dose. Then she is so grateful, and I breathe a sigh of relief.

Then there's Archie Bannister. He's another patient I inherited, this time from a colleague in my practice who retired. We all knew our retired colleague was a heavy opioid prescriber, but he was an excellent doctor, and his patients adored him. Of course, not all his patients were on opioids. But when he retired, suddenly there were 23 patients who were on very high doses of opioids to distribute between the 4 of us in the practice. Because of the opioid epidemic, and the 2016 Centers for Disease Control and Prevention guideline for prescribing for chronic pain, none of us were comfortable continuing the high-dose opioids, and so began an out-and-out war with many of these patients. Archie was one of these patients. Fifteen years ago, when he was 24, he injured his shoulder at work and subsequently underwent open shoulder surgery. He has been on opioids and has not worked since his injury. I know my job is to try to convince him that the opioid dose he is taking is unsafe, and probably not helping his pain much anyway. But he is convinced it is helping. He has been on it for years, and he has never had a problem with taking his medications as directed. So why take away the only thing that helps him get through the day? I spent 3 appointments trying to persuade him that he'd be better after a taper, but to no avail. In the end, I told him I would only continue to prescribe opioids if he tapered, so I started a slow taper. That was 4 visits ago, and every visit since then has been a battle. He used to be able to walk the dog, and now he says he can't even dress himself. He thinks I am treating him poorly and unfairly.

Then there's Joe Bolton. He's 28, and when he first became my patient, he was 19 and didn't have a pain problem. But lately he has become a frequent visitor in the clinic, complaining of pain in the groin, pain that becomes almost unbearable during intercourse. Other than groin pain, he is healthy, single, works as a nurse in a psychiatric hospital, and lives with his girlfriend. I have tried everything to try to help him, including the gamut of non-opioid pain medications and physical therapy, including heat and transcutaneous electrical nerve stimulation (TENS). I sent him to the pain clinic in town, which is run by a group of anesthesiologists based in the local surgicenter. They did a lot of diagnostic tests, including diagnostic nerve blocks and magnetic resonance imaging, but they couldn't find a treatable lesion, so their recommendation was to carry on with what I had been recommending. He is becoming increasingly socially withdrawn, is having difficulty sleeping, and has begun to talk about giving up work because the pain and insomnia make him so fatigued that he sometimes feels unable to cope. His girlfriend, frustrated, is threatening to move out. I don't know what else I can do other than a trial of opioids, which I'm trying to avoid because his age puts him at high risk of abuse. I get that sinking feeling every time he comes into the office because he is so distressed and frustrated with me.

Perhaps my most challenging patient is Susan Agasi. She comes in every week with her multiple medical problems. At 56, she has morbid obesity, sleep apnea, diabetes, hypertension, peripheral neuropathy, fibromyalgia, endometriosis, widespread joint pain, and headaches. She uses a wheelchair. She has not been a compliant patient, with poor self-care for most of her chronic illnesses. Over the years her medication requirements have gone up and up, so she now takes 13 medications altogether, including a high-dose opioid and a benzodiazepine, which we know is unsafe. I agreed to take her on after she fired one of the other doctors in our group. We had a group conference about how we should approach her, and decided we had to present a united front: She needed to come down on her opioid dose. She is very resistant to this, and every visit is a battle. We have offered Suboxone as an alternative to tapering, but she refuses to take a drug for "addiction" when she is not addicted. Every visit, her pain is worse, and sometimes she says she just can't manage the next-lower dose. So rather than argue, I kick the dose decrease down the road, which lets me off that visit, but makes me dread the next visit even more.

And although Enola Awinita isn't at all confrontational, I still dread her visit. She is such a sweet and sad person. When she was 6 years old, she was involved in a car crash that killed both her parents and her brother and left her paraplegic. She was adopted by her uncle, but her uncle didn't understand the challenge he was taking on looking after a child with serious disability. Over the years (she is now 32), pain in her legs and back became her predominant medical problem. She did not build up strength in her upper body or learn to be independent. She became increasingly reliant on others to get her from bed to chair, which is where she spends most of her life. She never leaves the house other than for medical appointments, and she is despondent to the point of being suicidal. She still lives with her uncle, who is frustrated and angry, and who often lashes out at her for ruining his life. She has used opioids for pain control since she was 15. The doses escalated to the point that the doses were very high, but never enough. The pain specialists thought it would help to put in a spine pain pump so that she could get opioids through the pump at lower doses (opioids delivered spinally are effective at much lower doses). But even though that helped initially, over time it has not helped at all, and now, nothing seems to help. When she comes to the office, she weeps uncontrollably and begs me to help her die.

So, I am sitting in my office waiting for the first new patient to arrive, and the medical assistant comes into the room to tell me that the first patient canceled. I have an hour, and instead of getting on with charting, I start thinking about why I feel so uneasy. The most difficult problems patients bring to me are chronic pain problems. When it's a recent pain problem, I can usually help with simple commonsense remedies, like a short course of rest, nonsteroidal medications, and gentle restoration of movement. Sometimes primary disease management helps, with cases like arthritis or diabetes. Sometimes surgery helps, when there is a clear, persistent, and gross pathological lesion. But then there are the long-term pain cases like the 5 patients I am seeing today. Did I help them? Where did I go wrong? Sometimes these problems just seem overwhelming. I wonder whether we are making the problems worse instead of better. Nobody ever taught me in medical school how to manage these harrowing problems, and a lot of the postgraduate education I got was about not letting these patients suffer needlessly without opioids because of unfounded fear of addiction.

I have learned that even though opioids help a lot initially, the patients who end up taking them for years, like the 4 patients on opioids I'm seeing today, don't really do well. They still have severe pain, which speaks for itself, and they are generally disengaged with life, and unhappy. But the most important thing I learned is that my patients who end up taking opioids for years were often distressed *before* they started taking opioids, and even *before* they developed protracted pain. *This makes me think that I didn't address the root cause of their pain.* Instead, I gave them drugs that numbed everything, which initially felt good, but could only be sustained by giving more drugs. And the more drugs I gave, the more unhappy they became. I became wrapped up in the sadness of their lives, and desperately sought solutions because I didn't want to fail them. I promised them pain relief that I couldn't provide. I let them be passive recipients of treatments that didn't really help, instead of recognizing their underlying distress, and helping them address it. I fell into the role of all-powerful healer, a problem solver and a fixer. Now I realize that healing is a partnership, and only works if I can succeed in helping the patients take care of themselves.

I have 2 new patients today. I don't even know if they have a pain problem, but given the prevalence of pain, it's quite likely that they do, or that they will develop one at some point in their lives. What shall I do differently today that I might not have done yesterday? I need to address any medical problems; that's what I'm here for after all. But I think I'll spend most of today's visit getting to know my new patients as people. Maybe I'll use questionnaires to get a handle on their psychological profile, but mostly, I'll just talk to them. If they have chronic pain, we'll talk about that. If they have social and emotional problems, my first goal will be to address them. We'll talk about what I've learned about how pain is a person's protective response to injury. How sometimes we have medical treatments for the injury, but the person must be involved in changing the response. If a person is already taking opioids, we'll talk about the pain in their life, and postpone talking about the opioids for now. Eventually, though, because the *person* is better able to control the pain than the *drugs*, we'll talk about the drug use. I think the most important thing I have realized is that unless there is a fixable structural cause for the pain, I can't change the pain. What I can do is to engage the patient as a partner. Not easily done, I know that. I will need new skills in patient motivation and empowerment. I now know that trying to remove pain with drugs will ultimately work against the goal of pain relief and an active, enjoyable, and fulfilled life.

Now, all these thoughts about how I'm going to do a better job of managing my patients' pain brings me back to Joe. He's not on an opioid yet, but the temptation to start is certainly the elephant in the room at every visit. I think of the other 4 patients, who are doing poorly despite being on opioids. I think about the fact that because I practice in a large city, multidisciplinary pain clinics and addiction services are available for my patients if I am out of my depth. I know that a lot of doctors who practice in remote places can't even access those services, and maybe don't even have psychologists they can work with. But even though I have good pain, behavioral health, and addiction services available, the burden of care still lies with me. I am the person who has to manage the long-term consequences of my treatment decisions. I can't send my 4 opioid-treated patients to addiction services because they aren't addicted. Still, as a consequence of their long-term opioid use, they all have opioid dependence, which is a complex and serious disorder that stands in the way of them getting better and is very challenging for me to manage. The specialists they have seen have nothing else to offer.

Same for Joe. Despite a long search for a fixable cause of his pain, and despite the best non-opioid approaches we know, he is really no better off than my 4 opioid-treated patients. The pain is interfering with every aspect of his life, and he is on a downward spiral. The only thing left for him is opioids. But wait! Have I really gotten to grips with what might be behind his pain problem? Did I ever assess him for depression, anxiety, posttraumatic stress disorder, or catastrophizing? Do I know if he was sexually abused as a child or even as an adult? Do I know anything about his home environment, what he does all day, and what his relationship with his girlfriend is like? Maybe I have to go back to the drawing board and first get to the bottom of what has been going on in Joe's life, and then build a partnership with him that takes him on the long road to recovery. I know opioids aren't the answer. But what I do have to offer, my engagement with him, could change his life.

11
Epilogue: Patient's perspective
My name is Reggie Winston

My name is Reggie Winston. This is the story of my back pain. I am a mechanical engineer, and my life was going pretty good. I had my own plane that I used to fly my family to Baja for vacations and my buddies to Idaho for camping trips. I went spear fishing in Mexico and backpacking in the Wind River Range. I had been jogging off and on for 20 years. I kept a tight grip on myself: dessert only on the weekends and no more than 3 ounces of alcohol each night. Barb and I had been married about 25 years. Our two oldest kids had graduated from college and were out of the house. Our twins, Sally and Sherry, had just started community college nearby. That was when Barb told me she wanted a divorce. It was a shock, but not a surprise, if you know what I mean. We had been arguing about this and that for years. Barb could be careless and silly in a way that drove me crazy. The fact that she was a bleeding heart liberal didn't help either. So we argued a lot, but I thought we would just stay together because we had stayed together through the four kids and now it was going to be easier. But she said she just had to get away from me. I was driving her crazy with my "know-it-all" attitude and she didn't love me anymore. I argued and pleaded and tried to change her mind, but it didn't work. By age 52, I was divorced and living in an apartment on my own.

For a while, I was OK. Well, I was not really OK, but my back was OK. It was lonely, but I kept flying and jogging and backpacking. But in August while backpacking with my old friend Ted I slipped coming down a trail and fell hard onto my butt. I felt bruised but was able to walk out of there just fine. But over the next few days my lower back started to ache. After a week, it had gotten worse and spread into both my hips. I took some aspirin and just tried to keep going. For a while it seemed manageable, but it didn't go away. My internist suggested I take some Aleve, so I started taking that twice a day. I got some relief so that I could work, but my sleep started getting messed up. I got to sleep fine after my nightly screwdrivers, but then I started waking up with back pain. I couldn't get back to sleep for hours sometimes. This just made me mad. I couldn't understand why I couldn't sleep even though I was really tired. I would just lie in bed and watch the clock tick by 2 a.m., then 3 a.m., then 4 a.m. My back was worse than ever during the day and I starting missing some work. There was no way I could fly my plane.

So I went to my internist and told him he had to do something to fix my back. He did a physical exam and found some numbness on the side of my thigh, so he ordered a lumbar computed tomography (CT) scan. The CT scan showed "degenerative disc and joint disease, with narrowing due to disc bulges at L4–5 and L5–S1." This sounded like a damaged spine to me, but my internist did not think I needed surgery. I was not ready to go home and just live with this awful back pain. So my internist referred me to a pain clinic for an epidural steroid injection. This was supposed to calm down the inflammation that might be driving the pain. That made sense to me, so I said, "Let's do it." And it worked like a charm. I felt great and started jogging and sleeping again. But it only lasted for a few months. Then I started waking up in the middle of the night again. And I felt too tired and sore to jog. I was pissed. I went to my internist and complained that his recommended treatment hadn't worked as promised. He explained that sometimes it took more than one steroid injection to get the inflammation and pain controlled for good. He sent me back to the pain clinic, where I got another epidural steroid injection. I got relief again, but this time it only lasted for a month. Now I really didn't know what to do. I had started dating one of the professors at the community college that my twin daughters went to. But since my back had gone out again, I was no fun and she didn't want anything to do with me. This added to my misery and bad attitude. I went back to the pain clinic doctor and asked what more he could do. He said we could do a third steroid injection. He offered me a bigger dose of steroid and said that might give me a longer period of relief. At that point, I was ready for any relief and said, "Go ahead." As you might be able to guess, I did not get much out of the third injection. Within weeks, my back pain was as bad as ever. I was not sleeping and more pain was running down my legs. I was unable to concentrate on work and was irritable with everybody.

I went back to my internist and asked him to do something. At this point, it had been a year since the back pain started. "Fix me" is what I said. I thought there must be something badly broken in my back. That is what it felt like. Machines don't just stop working unless a part breaks. So my internist ordered magnetic resonance imaging (MRI) of my back, which he said was more sensitive than the CT scan. The MRI showed a herniated disc pressing on my right L5 nerve root. Though I was having pain in both legs, my internist thought this might be the cause of my pain, so he sent me to a spine surgeon. The surgeon recommended a L5–S1 fusion where they remove the herniated disc and fuse the vertebral bodies above and below. The surgeon called this the "definitive fix" for problems at that level because it didn't just snip away at the disc or make more room for it, but removed it and fused the bones so there could be no more disc problems. I said OK because I was ready for something definitive. I wanted to be relieved of this pain once and for all.

The surgery went well. He got the disc out and fused L5 to S1 using a piece of bone from a cadaver. After surgery, the pain was better. At least the leg pain was better, and I could sit longer. My sleeping was better and my mood improved. I could do some work. I was doing some walking. After a few months, I felt confident enough to take my plane out for a spin. It was an easy short flight in good weather. But as I was landing, I hit a downdraft and bounced pretty hard on the runway. The plane's shock absorbers absorbed the impact, so the plane was not damaged. But my back was tweaked and went into spasm. I struggled to get out of the plane and walk back to my car. A feeling of doom overcame me. What would I do now?

My internist ordered another MRI. The fusion looked solid and there were no other ruptured discs. Everything looked OK, or at least what would be expected for someone facing his 54th birthday. My internist said there was no reason for more surgery. "So what then?" I replied. "You were supposed to fix me." I was so mad. I felt like I had been cheated. The "definitive fix" was anything but. I was desperate for relief. I deserved relief. I demanded relief. My internist looked at me and shrugged his shoulders. He said he could give me some Percocets. These had 5 mg oxycodone with some Tylenol in them. When I took one of them, I experienced relief from my pain. But I also got relief from feeling trapped in my life, trapped with my back pain in an awful little box. I had hope for a good life again.

The Percocets let me go back to work. My colleagues were glad to see me after all I had been through. At night, after I had my vodka, I found that I needed a couple of Percocet to sleep through the night. This went pretty well for a couple of months. Toward the end of the third month, I found that I was running out of my Percocets early. I must have been taking more of them. I went into my internist and told him that the Percocets had been working great, but that I needed a few more to get me through the month. I told him this was essential for me to be able to work. He said that since I was taking the Percocet around the clock it would be safer and more convenient if I took OxyContin because I only needed to take it twice a day. That seemed fine to me. He prescribed 20 mg in the morning and 20 mg in the evening.

This made things good again. I was able to work and even had a little energy to see friends. I met a nice woman, Vicki, through one of my work friends and we started dating. We would go out for dinner and drinks once or twice a week. After a few months I was back to working full-time, but I noticed that my morning pill would not hold me all day. I had some left-over Percocet, so I took some of those to help me sit through a stressful staff meeting or get a project finished on deadline. Sometimes I would take an extra Percocet at night if I thought I was going to have trouble sleeping. When I saw my internist, I told him I needed an occasional Percocet for when the pain broke through the OxyContin. He said he was familiar with breakthrough pain from his training in cancer pain management and gave me some Percocet to use only when I really needed it.

This combo worked really well to keep my pain level down and let me do what I wanted to do. I was able to work all day at my job and still feel good enough to have fun with Vicki. I took my OxyContin in the morning and evening, and carried some Percocet in my pocket for when I needed pain re-lief. Vicki was a lot of fun. She taught me how to rollerblade down the prom-enade by the beach. We would head out after work and then get dinner and drinks somewhere along the way. Things had been going great for months when we ran into Bruce at one of the restaurants. It was immediately clear that Bruce and Vicki knew each other, but that I was not supposed to know about Bruce and he was not supposed to know about me. To skip the yelling and just give you the bottom line, Vicki had been dating Bruce for about as long as she had been dating me. She didn't even feel that she should apologize about it, explaining that we weren't married. I was outraged and told her to f*** off.

When I got home, I was still in a rage. I knew I wouldn't be able to get to sleep and I had an important work presentation in the morning. I decided to take a couple of Percocet with my OxyContin so that I would be sure to sleep and be ready for my meeting. What I forgot is that Vicki and I had had a bit more to drink than usual. I did get to sleep, but I did not wake up in time for my meeting. In fact, I may not have woken up at all if my daughter Sally had not come by to pick up a wetsuit she was borrowing from me. It was 10 a.m. and I was blue and barely breathing. Sally could not wake me up. She called 911. The medics gave me some Narcan in my nose and I sat right up, coughing and sputtering. They took me to the hospital where I was diagnosed with an opioid overdose. I couldn't believe it. I told Sally, "This only happens to heroin addicts." Sally said, "You have been out of control for months. Sherry and I have been worried about you. We tried to talk to you, but you were having too much fun with Vicki. You were so happy to have your pain under control that you could not hear about anything else."

I did not know what to say. I had been taking my Oxys and my Percocets as they were prescribed. I was not an addict. It is true that I was not supposed to be drinking while I was taking them. But I was not drinking any more than I had been for years. I was never drunk. Sally said, "Maybe you weren't drunk, but you had become a different person, hiding behind those pills. Sherry and I could not talk to you about anything that mattered. It was like you were on a different emotional planet." Right then and there, I resolved to get off the pills and the booze.

But getting sober was easier said than done. I tried to quit everything all at once, but I went into terrible withdrawal and had a seizure. I was admitted to the hospital, where I was put on some Librium to cover the alcohol withdrawal and gradually weaned from that. I was discharged on tapering doses of opioids. I tried to follow the plan to taper off over a month or so. But my pain and insomnia and anger returned in a way I could not manage. My internist arranged for me to be admitted to an inpatient pain rehabilitation program, where they worked to get you off opioids and taught you other pain control strategies. I was in there for 4 weeks. And I did get off my opioids. My twins said I seemed like my old self.

My back pain never went away completely in the rehab program and as soon as I got home, it started getting worse. I did not know what to do. I went to my internist, who recommended a pain psychologist, Dr. Fitz, who had helped some of his other patients. There is no way that I would have gone to a psychologist before my surgery, but at this point, I was willing to try anything. Dr. Fitz said she could teach me some skills to help me better manage my pain on my own. Luckily, I had been an active person all my life, so I was eager to get back to doing more. The relaxation training or meditation was another matter. I didn't want to focus on my pain and I couldn't see how focusing on it would make it any better. I much preferred distracting myself by imagining I was at a beach or in the mountains. But that only worked for a short time and I couldn't do anything else while I was going on a vacation in my mind.

Dr. Fitz said that my rejection of my pain could be the core of my problems. I couldn't be at war with my pain and at peace with myself. She told me I had to change my relationship with my pain. "Pain acceptance" is what she called it. I didn't like the idea. It felt like admitting defeat to me. Fighting pain made more sense to me than accepting it. But she urged me to try just studying my pain without judging it right away. I was supposed to study it like a scientist, like it was a planet in outer space. This was very odd, but interesting. The pain did seem different when I was studying it like that. Instead of getting stronger when I was looking right at it, it got fuzzier. The boundaries between it and my other experiences, and between me and it, got blurry. Ironically, studying my pain like this became a way for me to get a break from my pain. But when I wasn't studying it, it was the same old pain.

Dr. Fitz said that we may have to look beyond my pain to other sources of hurt in my life. That struck me as a bunch of psychobabble that I would have laughed off years before. But I liked Dr. Fitz and she had taught me some useful things, so I kept listening. She asked me, "What is the most hurtful experience you have ever been through?" I immediately replied, "Getting divorced from Barb." She asked me to tell her the story of my divorce. I told her about how I had been blindsided by her asking for a divorce, just as we were getting the last kids out of the house, just as things were going to get a lot easier. I told her how angry I still was about this. It seemed unfair. I had been faithful and a good provider for many years. And then she threw me out.

"How painful that must have been . . . and must still be," said Dr. Fitz.

I was very surprised that I teared up at that point, something that I never do.

"Yes, I am still not over it. But I try to put it out of my mind and get on with my life."

"That hasn't worked too well, has it?" Dr. Fitz asked me.

"No, it hasn't," I replied, with some more tears. She said that the pain from the divorce was real pain, important pain, and that it was related to the pain in my back. I was carrying my pain with me. To get rid of my pain, she explained, I needed to drop my sense of being a victim. I needed to drop my long-nourished sense of anger at Barb. But I felt entitled to that anger, because she had done me wrong. Dr. Fitz said she did not think I could get rid of my pain without getting rid of my anger.

Later that week, I was out for a Mexican dinner with Sally and Sherry. I asked them whether I seemed angry most of the time. They looked at each other and said nothing. I said I would really like to know. They said, "Yes, you have always had anger right under the surface. But it got much worse after your divorce from Mom." That was a year ago. Since then, I have been doing a lot of expressive writing with Dr. Fitz. I have been working toward forgiving Barb. Dr. Fitz assures me that it is the path out of my pain, but it is the hardest thing I have ever done. But my back is feeling better.

Index